Assessment and Intervention in Geropsychiatric Nursing

Assessment and Intervention in Geropsychiatric Nursing

Celeste A. Dye, R.N., Ph.D.
Professor
Chairman of Graduate Studies
Director of Research
School of Nursing
University of Hawaii
Manoa, Hawaii

Grune & Stratton, Inc.

(Harcourt Brace Jovanovich, Publishers)
Orlando   San Diego   New York
London   Toronto   Montreal   Sydney   Tokyo

Library of Congress Cataloging in Publication Data

Dye, Celeste A.
    Assessment and intervention in geropsychiatric
nursing.

    Includes bibliographies and index.
    1. Geriatric psychiatry.   2. Psychiatric nursing.
3. Geriatric nursing.   I. Title.   [DNLM: 1. Aging—
nurses' instruction. 2. Mental Disorders—in old age.
3. Mental Disorders—nursing. WT 150 D995a]
RC451.4.A5D94   1985   618.97′689   84-25185
ISBN 0-8089-1712-9

Grune & Stratton, Inc.
Orlando, FL 32887

Distributed in the United Kingdom by
Grune & Stratton, Ltd.
24/28 Oval Road, London, NW 1

Library of Congress Catalog Number 84-25185
International Standard Book Number 0-8089-1712-9

Printed in the United States of America
85 86 87 88   10 9 8 7 6 5 4 3 2 1

To the memory of my brother
David Andrew Lombardi

Though humbled now, dishearten'd and distrest
Yet when admitted to the peaceful ground
With heroes, Kings and conquerors—I shall rest,
Shall sleep as safely, and perhaps as sound.

—*Philip Freneau*

Contents

Acknowledgments

A special debt of gratitude is owed to Susan J. Smith R.N., M.N., and Brenda Smith Jackson, R.N., M.S.N., C.C.R.N., for their research assistance in preparation of several chapters in this book.

Without the secretarial support and typing skills of Judy Tawater, this manuscript would not have been completed. Her ability to proofread and correct single-spaced copy replete with hieroglyphic notations is absolutely phenomenal, and for this we are most grateful.

For preparation of the original artwork, we are particularly indebted to the creative talents of Carol Hunter and Kathy Tull-Bowers.

Foreword

Experts from many fields have written about the growing population of the aged in our society. Each one has viewed the resulting dilemmas from the viewpoint of a particular specialty.

Celeste Dye would have done a service to the science of aging had she dealt just with the physical aspects, findings, and gaps in knowledge. A discussion of health and mental health issues would have contributed to general knowledge of the aging process. Each topic would have provided material for a suitable book. However, she has gone much farther. Building from her own background in nursing, rehabilitation, and psychology, she has gathered an impressive quantity of information into a volume characterized by a synthesis of findings, observations, and philosophy. To be able to meld scientific facts and thousands of pages of reading into a useful tool for the psychiatric nurse takes a special skill, one which Dr. Dye exhibits.

The author points out that to preserve the mental health of older people, we must preserve our own mental health. She also avows that while a philosophy of aging must be created, first we must redefine a philosophy of life. Threaded through all of the discussion of general issues are the examination and understanding of the human needs that underlie any assessment or decision-making procedures. Other authors have written about health requirements; many have taken up the psychological and psychiatric dilemmas, but this interweaving of fact and philosophy makes this book especially valuable for health care professionals who need the added insights, as well as for caring nonprofessionals who need the scientific information.

Bert Kruger Smith

Preface

The science of aging, like any science, begins in philosophy, and this book attempts to meld science and philosophy in an examination of mental health in old age. The book is written primarily for psychiatric nurses and other members of the health care team who provide direct service to the elderly. Yet because gerontology is a multidisciplinary field, every attempt has been made to make it useful to practitioners from other disciplines as well. Several themes recur throughout the book: the interaction of mind and body, the effect of environment on mental life, and the increasing need for a philosophical perspective of aging in a society buffeted by shifting values.

The text is divided into three parts. Part I examines normal aging by exploring various ways in which aging is defined, contemporary theories of aging, the relationship between aging, health and disease, and provides a review of biological changes. This is intended to update the knowledge base of the psychiatric-mental health professional. Part II introduces the assessment process through four major foci deemed important for the practitioner: assessment of mental processes, mind-body interaction, differential assessment of high-risk phenomena, and assessment of organic mental syndrome.

Part III offers guidelines for intervention. Individual, group, and family therapies are presented as examples of psychotherapeutic approaches suitable to the needs of this patient population. Because of the critical role that drugs play in their lives, chemotherapeutic guidelines are given substantial emphasis, with the hope of alerting the reader to the requirements and responsibilities involved in drug therapy with the older patient. The book ends with guidelines for sociotherapeutic intervention, addressing interventions that have been successfully implemented throughout public and private sectors, and raising crucial issues that await attention. Working with older adults is a challenging and vitalizing experience, and it is my hope that the reader will come to share this view.

PART I

Normal Aging

Aging is not one single process but many interacting processes. Each process encompasses multiple factors, such as degree of functional or structural change, or gradations of health and illness. The need for differentiation of the many types of factors is reinforced by a critical need for accuracy in assessment of mind–body interaction in the older adult.

The processes of aging are subtle and complex. They are essentially developmental in character and represent degrees of change—"change" is a word more genuinely representative of aging than the commonly used "decline"—taking place across time. Changes that begin at conception and continue throughout the life span are inevitable and irreversible. During infancy and childhood, development and maturation are measured with relative ease because of incremental growth spurts and plateaus that help establish normative data. Profiles of development in infancy and childhood are age-specific. During this period the continued interaction of time and maturation lead to adulthood because of the essentially anabolic character of aging. With adulthood and the attainment of maturity, however, aging processes assume an essentially catabolic character that leads to subsequent stages of senescence, and eventually to death. These latter stages of human development are not marked by easily measured, discrete intervals, so that adulthood and old age are represented more by estimated fluctuations in degree of change than by absolute, known values. In other words, all organisms decline as part of aging, but all organisms do not decline in the same manner or at the same rate. This raises several questions about how and why individuals differ so dramatically in aging. Why is decline so evident in certain individuals but not in others? Are there crucial changes due to normal aging processes and equally crucial changes due to disease that have escaped accurate clinical differentiation? How do structural, functional, temporal, or even environmental factors alter normal aging processes? Just what is "normal" aging?

Research findings have helped us move closer to an understanding of aging, but the field of gerontology in general and geropsychiatric nursing in particular is still in its infancy. Many of the questions are only partially answered. Discoveries made during recent decades have enabled us to reject notions of a single, common prototype for senescence. The robust physical and mental health of millions of older adults offers obvious evidence to the contrary. Their engagement in life, their competency, their vitality, and instrumentality make us wonder to what degree our perceptions have been colored by stigmas and stereotypes. As our understanding of aging increases we will be better able to clarify many of the misunderstandings that have prevailed for so long.

Part One of this book addresses these factors and separates those that may be considered "normal" in a healthy, functional sense from those associated with pathophysiologic change.

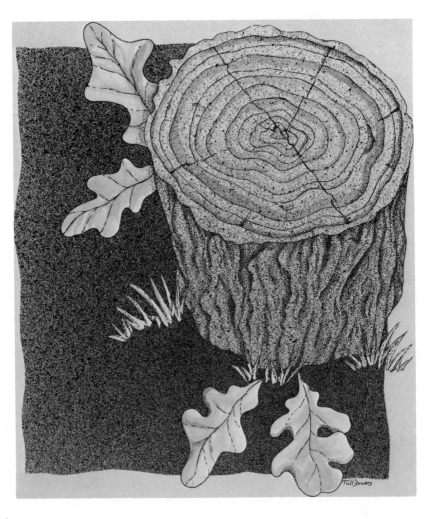

Chapter 1

Definitions of Aging

As the momentum of gerontological research continues, the number of persons presently age 40 or younger will reap significant rewards. As we learn more about aging processes, and the aging effects of disease, the coming scientific advances in life extension will increase the maximum life span for millions. The benefits of exercise, diet, and human interaction, and the known detriments of smoking, drugs, and inactivity, all publicized within the past two decades, will generate the healthiest old age ever known. We are witnessing the emergence of a new segment of society that, in its senescence, will be fitter, healthier, sounder of wind and limb, and more actively involved than ever before.

Chapter One examines the various ways in which aging has been defined, and concludes with a holistic and comprehensive perspective for contemporary nursing practice.

LEGAL AGE

Aging may be defined legally in several ways. Legal age is defined chronologically rather than either functionally or socially. There is a chronological determination of when one is an adult: at what age one may consume alcoholic beverages, drive a car, or leave school. Old age is also defined legally (if controversially) as the arbitrary attainment of age 65, when retirement becomes an occupational expectation if not a mandatory requirement (Cain, 1976). On the other hand, functional age would be determined by evidence of biological deterioration sufficient to interfere with the performance of work, and social age would be culturally determined by symbolic events such as the conferring of adulthood upon entrance into marriage. Chronological age has been widely used in the American legal system. The courts are presently faced with innumerable challenges to the legality of chronology as a definition suitable for mandatory retirement.

BIOLOGICAL AGE

A biological definition of age incorporates the developmental process, functional maturity, and chronology. Development continues in mammals usually until the cessation of long-bone growth. With the attainment of maturity developmental processes slow and gradually stop, while aging processes continue to accelerate. This acceleration of aging during postmaturity is characterized by decrements in function and in the organism's capacity to renew itself.

Biological definitions differ somewhat according to various authors. Some biological gerontologists have included in their definition the sum total of all changes in the species over the lifespan, with changes divided into developmental, maturational, and senescent phases. Any biological definition must include time–dependent changes occurring after maturity of size, form, or function is attained, with such changes distinctly differentiated from either daily, seasonal, or other biological rhythms. Biological definitions emphasize postmaturational change, particularly during senescence when structural and functional declines occur in unison.

SOCIOLOGICAL AGE

The social definition of age is culturally relative, so that "old age" is determined by the nature of aging and the role of age-related values within that culture. (Herskovitz, 1964). Various cultural standards determine that which is "old", and identify all meanings inherently associated with the word, so that its meaning varies considerably from one society and cultural frame of reference to another. In Plato's society the advantages of age far outweighed the disadvantages, and old age denoted wisdom in a culture where wisdom was venerated. In ancient India and China also, social values such as prestige and veneration of tenure graced the later years of life. According to Simone de Beauvoir (1973) the meaning or lack of meaning that old age assumes in any society puts the whole society to a test, since it is this that reveals the meaning or lack of meaning of the entirety of life leading up to it.

PSYCHOLOGICAL AGE

A psychological definition of age examines the adaptive capacities of individuals, and how well they adapt to changing environmental demands made upon them. Their capacity to adapt is then compared to the adaptive capacity of a comparable norm group. A psychological definition presupposes the availability of consistently revised normative or average data on specific variables. It is against these variables that legitimate comparisons may be drawn. Variables in the data profile may include biological (the health of organ systems such as the brain and cardiovascular system) as well as psychological (assessment of learning, intelligence, effective states, memory, cognition, emotion, psychomotor skills and motivation). Such data profiles have only recently been developed.

FUNCTIONAL AGE

Functional age is a relatively new, psychologically related construct that refers to the functional performance capability of an individual in comparison to others of matched age and potential. The construct of functional age, and the compilation of normative data regarding it require further refinement (Birren & Renner, 1977). Many factors, such as testing environment, test-taking behavior, and previous test scores affect functional performance capabilities of older subjects.

COMPREHENSIVE DEFINITION OF AGING

All previous definitions of aging have espoused a singular and somewhat selective view of aging. People were viewed as *either* legally (chronologically), socially, psychologically, biologically, or functionally aged, when in fact they are integrated, holistically complete and unique individuals. Many of the myths, stereotypes, and biases toward aging create misunderstanding. Hence it behooves us to consider aging with greater catholicity and attention to diversity.

The definition offered by Birren and Renner (1977) is fully comprehensive and rather widely accepted, perhaps because it includes biological, social, and chronological elements and allows for the inclusion of incremental as well as decremental changes in function across the life span. The authors refer to aging as the regular changes over time that occur in mature, genetically representative organisms living under representative environmental conditions. This definition encourages us to expand our perspective. This is vital if we are to comprehend the complex interactions taking place within the individual who is *simultaneously* a biological, chronological, psychological, functional and social organism.

"NORMAL" AGING

It has been very difficult to establish normative data on the healthy older adult. Interpretations of the mental and physical status of this age group have been based on data derived from young and middle-aged subjects.

Studies similar to the Duke University Longitudinal Study of Normal Aging (Palmore, 1970) must be undertaken to establish an appropriate data base (see Chapter 3). Too little is known of how the normal healthy elderly person differs from the normal healthy younger person. The goal of such investigations should be to differentiate specific ways in which the healthy elderly, who constitute 95 percent of America's aged, are different. What are the changes taking place in renal, cardiovascular, or endocrine systems, and how will they be affected by chronic illness? What are the normal emotional, motivational, and attitudinal changes taking place, and how will they predispose the individual to longterm illness?

We now know that we cannot refer to *the* aging process, since there are multiple processes at work that create progressive, inevitable changes in organ systems, which in turn alter general physiological functional capabilities. For instance, there is a gradual and irreversible decline with age in muscle strength, lung capacity, cardiac ability, kidney efficiency, and the speed with which sugar is metabolized. Yet, despite these declines, the built-in reserve capacity of the aged organism enables individuals to function amazingly well, and with little overall decline.

There is far greater variation in rates of aging among different individuals than was previously thought, and even greater differences in rates among different organs within the same individual. Part of the present dilemma of equivocal and inconclusive findings regarding rates of aging has to do with the discovery that the aged as a group are more heterogeneous than younger persons. This heterogeneity has served to illuminate the inappropriateness of norms derived from non-elderly subjects. ("Normal" refers to "average" or to those subjects falling two standard deviations above or below the mean on a bell-shaped distribution curve.) Problems arise when we realize that conditions of distinct abnormality for one aged group may be normal for another; for example decreased glucose tolerance or diminished ankle jerk reflexes are abnormalities or even diseases in the young, but are seen commonly in the aged. Does a high percentage of incidence in the elderly verify abnormality, or define normality?

"Normal" for most non-elderly groups implies the absence of disease, yet over 75 percent of all persons over 65 exhibit at least one chronic illness. The criteria by which "normal" is defined must be reexamined and broadened to include those aged persons of exceptional physical and mental health, those over 65 with at least one chronic illness, the high degree of heterogeneity of older subjects, and individual adaptability.

Aging is theoretically and clinically distinguished by four principle characteristics—it is universal, progressive, decremental, and intrinsic. Universality enables us to define aging as a normal phenomenon, similar to human growth and development. Future studies will show us how to articulate more precisely the difference between normal aging and that which is the result of disease.

SUMMARY

Normal aging is a phenomenon that incorporates temporal, physiological, psychological, social and biochemical elements. Aging is defined in various ways, with each definition suiting and providing direction for clinical practice and further research. A comprehensive definition is recommended for nurses who deal directly with the aged on a daily basis, since their ministrations involve the whole person during fluctuating states of illness and health. The normal elderly are presented as healthy, fulfilled individuals, while factors that both enhance and impinge upon their health are examined.

REFERENCES

Birren, J., Renner, V. (1977). Research on the psychology of aging: Principles and experimentation. In J. Birren & K. Schaie (Eds.), *Handbook of the psychology of aging* (pp. 3–38). New York: Van Nostrand Reinhold Co.

Cain, L. (1976). Aging and the law. In R. Binstock & E. Shanas (Eds.), *Handbook of aging and the social sciences* (pp. 342–368). New York: Van Nostrand Reinhold Co.

deBeauvoir, S. (1973). *The coming of age.* New York: Warner.

Herskovits, M. (1969). *Cultural dynamics.* New York: Alfred A. Knopf.

Palmore, E. (1970). *Normal aging.* Durham, NC: Duke University Press.

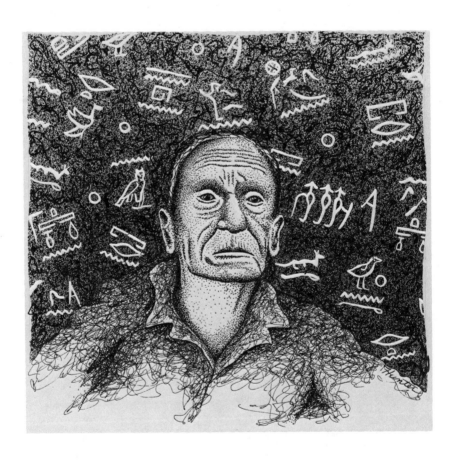

Chapter 2

Theories of Aging

Aging in humans is a conspicuous issue today because, unlike other species which remain unconscious of the aging process, humans are endowed with consciousness to perceive it, and intelligence sufficient to extend their life span. Man is seizing the opportunity to increase longevity and perpetuate his own species. Each organism's life span is predetermined by intrinsic biologic mechanisms. The kangaroo has a maximum life span of 20 years, the Capuchin monkey 40 years, the Asiatic elephant 70 years, and the Finback whale 80 years. On the other hand, the Mayfly lives out its entire adult life in a single day. Why are there such vast differences between and even within life species? Several theories are offered in this chapter, selected from among an increasing number of hypotheses.

HEREDITARY THEORIES OF AGING

Evolution Theory

The life span of humans exceeds the length that would be expected for mammals of our size. Sacher (1959) has proposed that this may be related to a greater brain weight to body weight ratio found in humans compared to other species. The greater size of the human brain may be a significant biological asset that contributes to longevity since, according to evolution theory, longevity is the result of a set of hereditary (genetic) characteristics that have evolved over centuries. Unlike other species, whose decline following the reproductive phase of life is very rapid, humans live for many years. The average woman today continues to live some four decades beyond her childbearing years. What evolutionary function could be served by this? Evolutionists have speculated that extended postreproductivity may have evolved as a means of protecting children and grandchildren, and could as well provide a means of transmitting vital knowledge to subsequent generations (Kimmel, 1980).

Genetic Program Theory

Genetic program theory holds that senescence is a product of a genetic program that has been exhausted. Each of us is born with a prearranged genetic plan. Our age changes are programmed much like a computer, from the moment of our conception to our maturity. Old age, according to this theory, is a condition in which the genetic program is completed, but the human organism, because of its great reserve capacities, is still functional. An analogy would be a powerless but still orbiting satellite (Comfort, 1979).

Counterpart Theory

In this theory aging is seen as the counterpart of early human development. Early development in this sense refers to stages of development prior to reproductivity. As the species evolved developmentally, certain traits and characteristics were subjected to the pressures of genetic selection. Characteristics that provided important adaptive capabilities early in life also contained negative counterparts that are manifested in senescence. Kimmel cites lack of cellular replacement of the central nervous system as an example. A species' ability to memorize and learn is greater with such cells, and therefore its chance for survival, but these same cells prevent the central nervous system from functioning indefinitely.

External Factors Theory

This theory examines behavioral, familial, environmental and biological elements that influence aging. Diet has been shown to extend the life span of laboratory animals, while cigarette smoking and obesity have been found to shorten it (Kimmel, 1980). The effects on elderly subjects exposed to radiation from nuclear testing and treatment for cancer have also been studied. Numerous investigations on animals have found correlations between radiation and shortened life span due to increases of various diseases, but no evidence has been found for acceleration of aging in humans. A related weakening of the human immune system, however, has been found. An additional aspect of aging is the force of mortality. The force or "risk" of mortality with advancing age is a concept developed by Gompertz (1825), who expressed as mathematical probability an exponential increase in mortality that transcended disease or increased life span. Kimmel has reported studies showing that if all cardiovascular and renal diseases were eliminated, only some 7.5 years would be added to the average life span, and if all cancer were eliminated only 1.5 years would be added. It is clear from these findings that force of mortality is still a viable concept, and that external factors play a significant role in the aging processes.

PHYSIOLOGICAL THEORIES OF AGING

Wear and Tear Theory

Proponents of the wear and tear theory believe that over time the human organism simply wears out. Nathan Shock (1962) has proposed that the diminution of organ functional reserve is a major component of aging by wear and tear, and indicates not that the body is unable to adapt to stress, but that it is not always able to do so rapidly enough. Though the rate of organ system degradation differs considerably within the individual, and even within components of the same system, aging imposes a gradual, progressive deterioration of organs necessary to support life. A depletion of the body's natural organ functional reserves takes place. Factors that have been found to influence the degradation rate include the opportunity for the organism to restore physiological equilibrium by alternating work and stress with sufficient rest, exercise, and nourishment.

Homeostatic Imbalance Theory

Homeostatic imbalance theory examines the interrelationship between stress, homeostatic balance, and the liability of the aged patient to psychophysiological illness. It does not equate stress with aging, or attempt to establish a causative relationship between homeostatic imbalance and aging processes. Rather, it concerns the diminished physiological capabilities in the aged person as a suitable precondition for the initiation of aging processes.

Efficiency of homeostatic mechanisms is crucial to maintenance of physiologic balance in the body (for example in maintaining blood sugar levels and pH), but several studies of homeostatic regulation (Goldman, 1979; Kimmel, 1980; Selye, 1970) have shown that following periods of stress older subjects are far less able to restore normal physiological equilibrium than younger subjects. They are less able to maintain renal, thermal, or blood sugar homeostatis because in general their self-regulatory mechanisms have become less efficient. Stress is a major factor in homeostatic inefficiency and places the aged subject at considerable risk. Vulnerability is increased by inadequate monitoring of homeostatic balance, impaired endocrine responses, and decreased sensitivity to hypothermia. Stress of psychogenic as well as physiogenic etiology must be considered, since varied sources of psychological stress (discussed in Chapter 1) are being experienced by the individual who is already physiologically at risk.

Metabolic Waste and Cross-Linkage Theory

Metabolic waste products accumulate with age, and some scientists believe that the accumulation of this waste slowly impairs the function of the body's cells (Kimmel, 1980). Collagen and lipofuscin have been studied extensively, and both are believed to be involved in the more visible signs of aging. Both substances accumulate slowly, and both are thought to be eliminated even more slowly, if at all. Collagen buildup in the aged is thought to be at least partially responsible for the wrinkling of skin and the slower rate of wound healing. Lipofuscins accumulate in some nerve cells and produce pigmentation in these cells while causing a partial decline in cell function.

Concentrations of lipofuscin in cell cytoplasm have been found to be a generalized phenomenon in most postmitotic, non-dividing cells (cardiac, skeletal muscle, and neural), as well as in adipose tissue, the liver, and adrenal glands. Additional waste is accumulated as a result of improper calcium metabolism, a process which shifts calcium from bone to soft tissue, and leaves a subsequent brittleness of bone.

Cross-linking is the result of molecules within and without the cell linking into denser aggregates that impair normal cell function. It is more common in subjects with collagen formation. The development of these cross-linked, intertwined strands is being closely investigated, but there is little evidence to date that cross-linking is a cause of aging, and far more evidence that it may be no more than a symptom (Kimmel, 1980).

Autoimmunity Theory

The hypothesis that autoimmunine reaction is a cause of aging is now considered provocative, but not fully tenable (Adams, 1980; Carotenuto, 1980; Everitt & Huang, 1980). It was a hypothesis that lent itself to rigid experimental testing conditions, and data gained from these experiments may well generate subsequent hypotheses and methodologies that reveal aging etiology. The theory is important to any discussion of aging, however, because it does address secondary if not primary factors that influence aging processes, such as the increased risk of disease.

The thymus, master gland of the immune system, produces two types of lymphocytes to defend the body against invaders of internal or external origin. B cells attack invaders by production of antibodies, while T cells directly attack viruses and bacteria. T cells assist B cells by identifying invasive organisms among the body's own cells. The thymus begins to shrink at puberty, and by senescence is producing fewer and less efficient T cells. The number of B cells circulating in the bloodstream also decreases, resulting in a generalized decrease in the capabilities of the autoimmune system.

Immunologists have also shown that the autoimmune system can produce antibodies that attack substances that occur quite naturally within the body. These autoantibodies have been suggested as a possible cause of rheumatoid arthritis, systemic lupis erythematosus, Hasimoto's thyroiditis, and other diseases. Some investigators believe that these autoantibodies may cause aging, since the immunologic system becomes unable over time to differentiate normal from foreign proteins, resulting in an inadvertent destruction of normal proteins.

CELLULAR THEORIES OF AGING

These theories see aging as a symptom of the change in the size, number, and structure of human cells. In time there is an overall loss of cells as measured by organ weight, total cell count, and amount of potassium, DNA, intracellular water, and nitrogen. Postmitotic cells (those no longer capable of reproduction; primarily nerve and muscle) are not replaced when lost and their number decreases with age. Remaining cells demonstrate characteristic pigmentation within the storage granules of cell cytoplasm, structural distortion in the form of fragmented chromosomes, and reduced mitochondria (Kimmel, 1980).

Doubling Theory

It was thought originally that cells grown in vitro could, under favorable growth conditions, live forever. The implication was that cells could reproduce an infinite number of times, and that there was no intrinsic limit to life if conditions in vitro could be replicated in vivo. Studies conducted by Leonard Hayflick (1975) over a number of years, however, have revealed that a cell's replicative capacity, or number of doublings, is fixed by a biological clock. He found that human embryo cells always died after 50 doublings. He also found that cells have memories; when cell division was clinically interrupted by freezing and storage in liquid nitrogen for several years, it was found upon thawing that cells were able to resume doubling, and to continue until they reached their limit of 50 doublings.

DNA Repair Theory

A theory related to the doubling theory suggests that DNA, the master molecule of life, is constantly damaged by bombardment of ultraviolet light, a process requiring rapid enzymatic repair so that DNA may restore its information-carrying function (Finch & Hayflick, 1977). It is thought that a breakdown in the repair enzymatic system results in damaged DNA sending incorrect instructions to cells, which causes malfunctioning in cell activity.

Progeria, a rare disease in which aging processes are accelerated in children, is an example of such malfunctioning DNA transmission. Though they appear normal at birth, prior to adolescence progeric patients lose their hair, have thin bones, wrinkled skin, and cardiovascular disease, and by adolescence they exhibit the chronic illnesses of old age.

Error Catastrophe Theory

DNA is an essential source of genetic information for human development and function. The information encoded in DNA is conveyed through the synthesis of proteins, which are either enzymatic, regulatory, or structural. While DNA does not serve directly in protein synthesis, it acts as a template for the synthesis of messenger RNA in a process referred to as "transcription." The error catastrophe theory suggests that an impairment of RNA synthesis, causing improper transcription of information from DNA, leads to a catastrophe of errors that damage cell function and division. Errors accumulate in the amino sequences in proteins, particularly those affecting enzyme specificity required for protein synthesis, and this leads eventually to cell deterioration and death. Some scientists now believe that the greater the number of errors in macromolecular constituents the more rapid the accumulation of further errors (Finch & Hayflick, 1977).

Pacemaker Theory

Some gerontologists believe that a pacemaker mechanism in the brain triggers aging processes in much the same fashion that puberty and menopause are activated. Caleb Finch (1975) theorizes that neurohormonal events in the body are controlled by monoamine transmitters such as serotonin, dopamine and norepinephrine. He believes that since many hormonal systems are controlled by the nervous system, alterations of certain neurons in the ventral portion of the brain may regulate aging. Others (Adams, 1980; Carotenuto 1980; Everitt & Huang 1980) believe that the body's immune system rather than the brain is the pacemaker, but all agree that the role played by the central nervous system in activating aging processes is pivotal.

Free Radical Theory

Free Radical theory has as its central hypothesis the theory that free radicals, or unstable, highly reactive molecular endproducts of metabolism damage the cell's ability to function. Free radical damage to cells is offset by the body's production of scavenger enzymes called antioxidants, which search out free radicals and combine with them to prevent cellular damage. As people age, however, fewer antioxidants are produced. Free radicals can also be generated by chemicals found in food, tobacco smoke, and air pollutants. Dietary supplements containing substances having high antioxidant properties such as vitamins C and E and selenium are being tested as possible preventive measures.

PSYCHOSOCIAL THEORIES OF AGING

Disengagement Theory

Disengagement theory emerged from the early work of Cummings and Henry (1961). They studied healthy, white, middle-class Americans, and found that their ability to disengage from various life roles late in life enhanced that period for them. The theory posits a mutual withdrawal agreement between the elderly and society, one that is inevitable and gratifying for both. According to Cummings and Henry, the elderly must relinquish social status, positions of leadership, work, and familial roles in order to provide opportunities for younger individuals to assume roles they are no longer able to hold, and thus maintain society's equilibrium. This theory has fallen from favor in recent years. Critics have argued that it provides little more than a rationale for exclusion of the aged from the social mainstream, while denying them equity in the distribution of welfare and health care benefits. At present the theory may be considered a credible explanation of a social phenomenon that has existed for centuries, rather than an explanation of aging.

Activity Theory

This theory holds that superior adjustment to old age is made by persons who establish a high level of social activity in middle age and maintain that level into later life (Carnevali & Patrick, 1979). Social roles that are relinquished as the subject ages must be replaced with viable substitutes, since a high degree of social activity is proposed as central to high morale and life satisfaction. Participation in community life through organized groups is recommended to meet fundamental human needs for social interaction, and to prevent the deteriorative effects of isolation and withdrawal. The theory has been criticized for its value-laden premise that activity is unquestionably beneficial, and for its failure to address myriad variations in individual capacity for physical and mental activity that exist in highly heterogeneous populations.

Developmental Theory

Developmental theory perceives the aging processes as progress through a life cycle of developmental phases, which are characterized by specific normative conflicts and psychosocial tasks (Erikson, 1959). At each phase of development the individual is confronted by opposing forces, positive and negative, which must be synthesized for progression to continue. In late adulthood the crises involve generativity or the creative use of self, versus stagnation or the impoverishment of self.

In old age the dilemma is to reconcile the extent to which one has achieved integrity, or a sense of personal worth and uniqueness, with despair or a sense of personal loss and contempt (Dye, 1979). One cannot progress to a particular stage until the crises of the previous stages have been resolved. The theory also addresses the relationship between innate individual capacities and the expectations of others, and provides for interpretations of "successful" aging in terms of personally defined standards rather than those dictated externally.

An inherent danger lies not in developmental theory itself, but in its interpretations. Proponents often misapply the principles of emperical measurement, applicable to physical growth and development, to mental and emotional status, resulting in imprecise estimations of mental health. Precise measurements of despair, ego integrity, or generativity are not possible, since they are concepts defined culturally and therefore subject to considerable variation. The theory has, however, provided a fertile research laboratory for social and psychological gerontology, and will in all likelihood continue to do so well into the future.

Symbolic Interactionist Theory

Symbolic interactionist theory is based upon three basic tenets first proposed by Herbert Blumer (1969). These are as follows:

- individuals act toward things based upon the meaning such things hold for them
- the meaning of things is determined by the nature of social interaction with others
- meanings are modified by encountering things

According to symbolic interactionism, reality as a concept is constructed socially through an ongoing process of interpretation. Knowledge is "invented" as individuals determine what is true and real for them. The individual self both determines and is determined by interpersonal interaction. Social behavior involves a process of continual, creative change.

The symbolic nature of behaviors, events, circumstances and communication all influence the meanings and actions one experiences. For the aged the symbolic significance of things, people, and experiences, and the types of interaction encountered, all determine the nature of meanings derived, and resultant degrees of satisfaction felt. While the theory does not identify particular behaviors or experiences in old age, its emphasis upon socially constructed meaning and symbolic significance is evident, for example, in perceptions of the nursing home as a prelude to death, or a beneficent haven. The social context is crucial to any understanding of aging, since all values and meanings are dynamic rather than fixed or static. This theory is expandable, in that limitless variables may be included to study aging processes, and offers almost limitless opportunities for investigation to students of aging.

SUMMARY

A review of the theories presented here demonstrates the breadth of ideology regarding aging. Hereditary theories explain aging in terms of the evolutionary properties of the species, of genetic programs incorporated at conception which either run out or are manifested in senescence, and of variant factors that influence (yet do not determine) the length of life. Physiological theories range from views of man as a machine corroded by time, to a victim of biology assaulted by free radicals. The possibilities of homeostatic imbalance, accumulated waste, autoimmunity, finite DNA reproductivity, and pacemaker activation–regulation all offer exciting promise for research in the years ahead. The physiological perspective is fundamentally one of human aging as a biological phenomenon in search of causation. Psychosocial theories in contrast are descriptive rather than experimental and perceive aging from various phenomenological and ideological orientations.

REFERENCES

Adams, R. (1980). The morphological aspects of aging in the human nervous system. In J. Birren & R. Sloane (Eds.), *Handbook of mental health and aging* (pp. 149–160). Englewood Cliffs, NJ: Prentice-Hall.

Blumer, H. (1969). *Symbolic interaction: Perspective and method*. Englewood Cliffs, NJ: Prentice-Hall.

Carnevali, D., Patrick, M. (1979). *Nursing management for the elderly*. Philadelphia: J.B. Lippincott.

Carotenuto, R., Bullock, J. (1980). *Physical assessment of the gerontologic client*. Philadelphia: F.A. Davis.

Comfort, A. (1979). *The biology of senescence* (3rd ed.). New York: Elsevier.

Cummings, E., Henry, W. (1961). *Growing old*. New York: Basic Books.

Dye, C. (1979). Developmental reactions in old age. In M. Kalkman & A. Davis (Eds.), *New dimensions in mental health psychiatric nursing* (5th ed.). New York: McGraw Hill.

Erikson, E. (1959). Identity and the life cycle. *Psychological Issues, 1*(1).

Everitt, A., Huang, C. (1980). The hypothalamus, neuroendocrine and autonomic nervous systems in aging. In J. Birren & R. Sloane (Eds.), *Handbook of mental health and aging* (pp. 100–133). Englewood Cliffs, NJ: Prentice-Hall.

Finch, C. (1975). Neuroendocrinology of aging: A view of an emerging area. *Bioscience, 25,* 645–650.

Finch, C., Hayflick, L. (1977). *Handbook of the biology of aging.* New York: Van Nostrand Reinhold Co.

Goldman, R. (1979). Aging changes in structure and function. In D. Carnevali & M. Patrick (Eds.), *Nursing management for the elderly* (pp. 53–80). Philadelphia: J.B. Lippincott.

Gompertz, B. (1825). On the nature of the function expressive of the law of human mortality on a new mode of determining life contingencies. *Philosophical Transaction of the Royal Society (London), Series A. 115,* 513–585.

Hayflick, L. (1975). Cell biology of aging. *Bioscience, 25,* 629–637.

Kimmel, D. (1980). *Adulthood and aging.* New York: John Wiley & Sons.

Sacher, G. (1959). Relation of lifespan to brain weight and body weight in mammals. In E. Wolstenholme & M. O'Connor (Eds.), *CIBA Foundation symposium on the life span of animals.* London: Churchill.

Selye, H. (1970). Stress and aging. *Journal of the American Geriatrics Society, 18*(9), 669–690.

Shock, N. (1962). The physiology of aging. *Scientific American, 206*(1), 100–110.

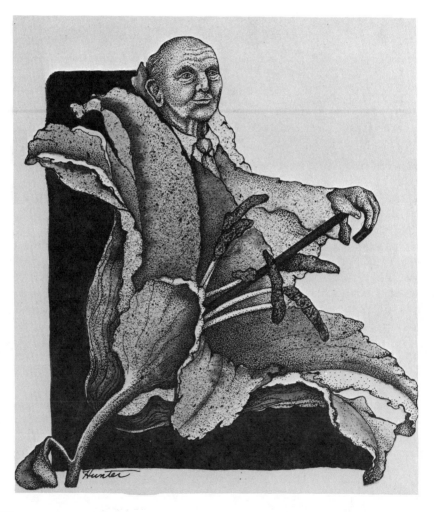

Chapter 3

Health, Aging, and Disease

The Duke Longitudinal Study of Normal Aging resulted in the generation of 48 tentative hypotheses concerning the normal aged person living in the community (Palmore, 1970). Some of the findings of this investigation are presented here, to illustrate the many ways in which health is possible in senescence.

The physiological, social, and psychological status of 256 subjects was analyzed over a period of almost 14 years. Various methods were used to collect data, including physical assessment techniques, direct questioning, clinical depth interviews, and both projective and objective psychometric testing. While half of the aged subjects exhibited some degree of decreased physical capacity the remaining half did not, and other subjects even demonstrated significant physical improvement over time. Subjects from a lower socioeconomic status exhibited more limited physical functioning than those from a higher socioeconomic status. The physical capacity of these normal individuals did not differ according to sex or race. Over one third of the subjects were found to have one or more neurological impairments and most had either skin problems and one or more symptoms of vascular disease.

NORMAL PSYCHOLOGICAL FINDINGS

Subjects reacted more slowly to interview and testing instructions, but it was found that reaction time could be improved with practice. Greater individual differences in reaction time, and slower responses to testing conditions associated with less physical exercise were also found. Intelligence was shown to be stable across time, and performance on projective tests was shown to relate more to intelligence level than to age. Intelligence was also shown to be unimpaired by cardiovascular disease.

Hearing loss was found to impair emotions, vocabulary and perception more than visual loss. Subjects tended to express less emotion than younger persons but considerably more than ill persons. They perceived auditory stimuli as well as younger individuals. In general, memory recall was poorer than that of younger persons, but as good as the young when examination content held strong meaning for them.

Successful marriages were characterized by husbands who were older than, and of equal or superior mental ability to, their wives, by frequent sexual activity, and by the absence of mental illness. Most subjects with children lived apart from them but maintained affectionate and to some extent dependent ties with them. Men exhibited greater sexual interest and activity than women. Half of the men aged 72–77 remained sexually active, as did a fourth of those over 78. The majority of subjects experienced some decline in sexual interest and activity during the 14-year period, but a substantial minority maintained stable interest and activity levels, and some even experienced increases.

Disability caused a decline in social activity but was not found to influence satisfaction in life. The primary factor influencing attitude and social activity level was socioeconomic status. Patterns of attitude and social activity remained stable across time, but declining physical activity was found to impose a decline in life satisfaction. Subjects' appraisals of their own health were found to be realistic and consistent. Hypochondriasis was more often associated with younger, less active females of lower socioeconomic status. Identification with an age category (young, middle-aged, old, etc.) had no relationship to attitude or activity, but was related to chronological age rather than any other factor. Two-thirds of the subjects identified themselves as "old." Black subjects and those in poor health identified themselves as "old" most often, and black subjects found more advantages to old age than did white subjects.

Concern for the future and fear of death were minimal, and were associated with little religious reading, little belief in life after death, depression, and lower intelligence. The most important factors found to relate to longevity were health, mental abilities, and satisfying social roles.

The findings of this study are interesting in several ways. First, they demonstrate that the normal elderly are able, even in the presence of disease and diminished physical capacity, to retain and to use a high degree of functional autonomy. Over a 14 year period their energy levels declined, their visual and auditory actuity became less sharp, and moderate degrees of debilitating disease appeared. We might easily have expected subjects of such advanced age to perform less well in interview and testing situations. Their stamina is impressive.

Second, the findings fail to support commonly accepted stereotypes of old age; instead, they seriously refute them. Intelligence appears to remain stable over time. Also, the elderly appear able under rigid testing conditions to compensate for sensorimotor deficits. Though reaction time is slower, with practice the elderly are able to improve performance more than younger subjects. In addition, the myth of asexuality in senescence is disproven by the fact that sexual interest and activity, considerably higher than expected, remains evident well into the seventh decade of life.

Third, rather than believe themselves socially devalued or psychologically degraded by their present life circumstance, the normal aged person presented a healthy, positive outlook toward life. Each subject's patterns of attitude (which might have been influenced by the negative attitudes of others) and social activity remained stable over several decades. Satisfaction with life remained high until affected by declining physical and social activity. There is obviously a healthy, resilient optimism in their strong desire to remain not only active but directly involved in satisfying social roles. The fact that the primary influence on their activity and attitude is socioeconomic rather than psychosocial says more about prevailing economic, social welfare, and health care conditions than it does about the psychology of aging. The findings generally make us question many of the assumptions about the inevitability of decline in old age, and about uniformity in rates of decline. Previously unexamined compensatory mechanisms appear to be available to individuals as they age, and if these subjects are any example, they seem to be able to utilize these mechanisms with adroitness and skill.

DISEASE

Aging changes per se are dependent upon many many factors, not the least of which is the current definition of disease. Not too many years ago arteriosclerosis was considered a natural manifestation of aging, because its incidence was greater among older persons and because clinical profiles showed its greatest severity among certain persons of advanced age. Today arteriosclerosis is considered a complex metabolic disorder and is defined as a disease. As scientific advances offer clarification of "disease" versus "aging" we will be able to move beyond present ambiguities and imprecision.

Aging processes and disease processes are complexely intertwined, and Hans Selye's (1970) belief that aging is the result of disease-induced, accumulated deficits may well be proven correct. For the present our knowledge is limited to findings that show a strong, positive correlation between the effects of disease on the effects of aging, with the effects of one compounding the other. For example, as physical capacity declines even moderately, awareness of it induces a disturbance of emotional equilibrium. As emotional equilibrium is unbalanced even moderate sensory losses in hearing and vision assume greater importance. The combined effect of sensory, emotional and physical deficit is greater than any single component, and often predisposes the accident-prone elderly to injuries that will take longer to heal.

Disease is an important consideration in aging because the effects of aging alone may be relatively minor while the imposition of disease may introduce a wide range of consequences. Even a mild degree of disease may initiate broad systemic effects because of the various organic and systemic changes taking place. Acute illnesses are more common to younger age groups and the incidence of acute disease tends to decrease with age. The incidence of chronic illness, in contrast, escalates markedly with chronological age. Artereosclerosis, cardiovascular disease, respiratory disease, hypertension, arthritis and rheumatism are more common chronic diseases found in the aged. The chronic nature of these diseases exerts a profound psychological, social and economic effect. Studies of chronicity (Kalish 1975; Kart & Metress, 1978; Kimmel 1980) have shown that many of the major psychological problems of aging are associated with long-term physical illness. Awareness of physiological change may easily predispose individuals to preoccupation with their health and with feelings of depression. A return to former levels of wellness is no longer possible, and the mourning of lost vitality is commonplace.

Economic consequences of chronic disease include an increase in expenditure for health care, and in number of office visits for treatment. Those over 65 tend to have medical expenditures 3.5 times that of individuals under 65. Socioeconomic status is also a salient issue. While arthritis, which was prevalent among over one third of the respondents in the Duke study, was not found to be related to socioeconomic status, most other common chronic diseases were. Arteriosclerosis, cardiovascular disease, hypertension, and respiratory disease were all observed more frequently in the lower socioeconomic group. Persons in the higher socioeconomic group showed less disability, and it is probable that chronicity is a cause as well as a consequence of lower income.

The number of visits to physicians increases with age. Figure 3-1 shows that for the period between 1968 and 1969 the number of visits increased successively with age. According to the National Center for Health Statistics (U.S. Department of Health, Education, and Welfare, 1978) the number of physician contacts has increased in recent years for all age groups so that by 1976 visits for persons 65 and over had increased to 6.7 per year. Women show a slightly greater tendency to seek medical treatment than men. This may be attributable to a machismo ethic in males denying illness rather than greater incidence of illness in females. Women are also less likely to be hospitalized than men. Again, masculine mores may be producing negative attitudes toward illness and early help-seeking behavior in men.

Chronic impairments, such as reduced hearing, visual loss and blindness, loss of teeth, loss of mobility and restricted activity, curtail one's

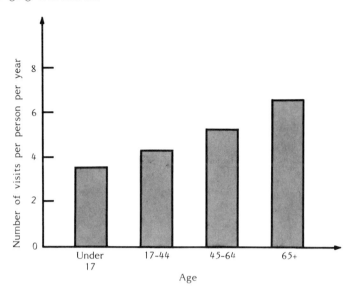

FIGURE 3-1. Number of physician visits per person by age, United States. 1968–1969. (U.S. Department of Health, Education and Welfare, 1972).

natural life style, yet for more than 80 percent of those over 65 no impairment has been found to limit function in major activities. Physical activity has been shown to decrease generally with age, and this may provide a significant variable for future research on aging and motor performance. Hypokinetic disease (physical and mental changes induced by inactivity) is present even in younger subjects, suggesting that regular, physical exercise is vital to everyone's health. Three weeks of bedrest have been shown to induce decline in maximal cardiac output, maximal ventilatory capacity, oxygen consumption, and active tissue mass even in young persons. Decline in certain physiological variables significant to human performance have been found to be more highly related to decreased habitual activity level than to age itself. Hence great emphasis must be placed on initiating and maintaining programs of regular physical exercise. (Goldman, 1979; Kart & Metress, 1978; Kimmel, 1980).

CAUSES OF DEATH

The major causes of death in the elderly population include heart disease, cancer, cerebrovascular diseases, influenza, pneumonia, arteriosclerosis, diabetes, accidents, and chronic obstructive pulmonary disease (COPD). More than 80 percent of the deaths in this age group are caused by cardiovascular disease, cancer, and accidents, and the death rate from heart disease is more than three times greater than that from any other cause. The rate for women is lower than that for men from almost all causes. Racial differences are evident in a death rate for blacks that is almost twice as high as for whites from renal infections, diabetes, cerebrovascular disease, arteriosclerosis, influenza and pneumonia. Such racial differences exist for individuals in the 65-74 year old age group, but thereafter a reversal in life expectancy becomes apparent with blacks over 80 living longer than whites. The reasons for this phenomenon are unclear, and considerable research remains to be done. It has been speculated that reporting errors in census data and differential demographic variables such as age, occupation, education or income may account for some of the difference. In addition, data on autopsies are often inaccurate. Autopsy rates decrease as the age at death increases, due probably to the more common expectation of death in old age. Few requests for post-mortem examination are made and fewer examinations conducted on the aged, resulting in less valuable information on normal and abnormal changes at the time of death. Vital information about normal aging changes and pathophysiologic dysfunction is forfeited by this practice, and interest in obtaining permission for autopsies needs to be generated.

HEALTHY AGING

Normal aging is confounded by chronic disease and its secondary consequences. Changes in drug detoxification, blood flow to the liver, renal decrements, and metabolic rates in later life, in conjunction with inadequately trained health personnel, leave this whole area of age–change versus disease–change insufficiently studied and open to conjecture. Birren, Butler, Greenhouse, et al. (1963) undertook an investigation that produced some promising results. They studied a sample of 47 men aged 65-91, all in apparently excellent health. Extensive in-depth examinations, which included multiple medical, social, psychological and physiological variables, revealed that there were actually two distinct groups being studied; Group A whose subjects were in optimal health and Group B whose subjects were asymptomatic but discovered to have mild, subclinical diseases. On all variables studied Group B subjects performed less well than subjects in Group A. An integrative effect appeared to be reinforcing or canceling the effects of various factors in a complex interdependency. In the presence of even asymptomatic disease the dependency of psychological capacity on physiological status was increased; i.e., dependency on mind in the mind–body equation was heightened by the introduction of disease. Hence disease became the third variable in the aging–psychophysiology formula, suggesting that even mild illness may force stronger correlations between mind, age, and body than previously believed.

An eleven year follow-up study of the same subjects by different investigators revealed that 70 percent of Group B subjects had not survived while 63 percent of Group A subjects had. Two early predictors of mortality, cigarette smoking and organization of daily behavior, when combined correctly predicted 80 percent of survivors and nonsurvivors. Survivors were found to exhibit very little change with age, but correlations between psychological and physiological status were even more pronounced. Kimmel (1980) has interpreted the findings in the following manner. Changes frequently attributed to aging might well be considered the result of disease; in the absence of disease there are important age-related changes in physiology but less impairment than is commonly believed; age-related changes alone seem to be relatively minor but may increase vulnerability to stress and disease.

HIGH RISK FACTORS

Some of the common phenomena that present high risk problems for the normal aged include loneliness, depression, multiplicity of loss and perception of powerlessness in society. Loneliness is related to attrition in the number and types of relationships available to the elderly, as well as to their capacity for the establishment of new ones. It is often caused by geographic isolation, a language barrier, ethnic and cultural impediments, illness, stereotyping, or personal life-style. Loneliness is not simply a desire for any type of company, but a desire for certain forms of relationship. These highly specific forms of relationship must be identified so that steps can be undertaken to foster their development.

Depression, like loneliness, has been shown to· seriously affect the homeostatic equilibrium of the patient. If untreated it leads to catastrophic decline and even to early death. Depression is the most serious mental problem in old age and its incidence (estimates range from 10–65 percent of persons over 65) varies by age, time of onset (usually in the fifth and sixth decades of life), and by complicating, intervening variables such as organic brain damage or secondary effects of disease. Somatic effects often result from hypochondriacal symptoms that characterize the more common forms of depression in old age.

The stressors of late life that may alter normal homeostatic processes include the cumulative effects of diminished mobility, a gradual reduction in one's sphere of social influence, diminished sources of diversion that retain levels of interest and enthusiasm, diminished communication within a circle of close friends, fewer contacts with people in general, diminished resistance to disease and traumatic injuries, and diminished opportunities if not inclinations for sexual activity. Further, the gradual losses of youthful appearance, confidence in one's cognitive ability, and first-class citizenship

Table 3-1 Effect of External and Physiological Factors on Length of Life

Reversible		Permanent	
Comparison	Years	Comparison	Years
Country versus city dwelling	+5	Female versus male sex	+3
Married status versus single,		Familial constitutions	
widowed, divorced	+5	2 grandparents lived to 80	
Overweight		years	+2
25 percent overweight group	−3.6	4 grandparents lived to 80	
35 percent overweight group	−4.3	years	+4
45 percent overweight group	−6.6	Mother lived to age 90 years	+3
55 percent overweight group	−11.4	Father lived to age 90 years	+4.4
67 percent overweight group	−15.1	Both mother and father lived	
Or: an average effect of 1		to age 90 years	+7.4
percent overweight	−0.17	Mother lived to age 80 years	+1.5
Smoking		Father lived to age 80 years	+2.2
1 package cigarettes per day	−7	Both mother and father lived	
2 packages cigarettes per day	−12	to age 80 years	+3.7
Atherosclerosis		Mother died at 60 years	−0.7
Fat metabolism		Father died at 60 years	−1.1
In 25th percentile of		Both mother and father died	
population having		at age 60 years	−1.8
"ideal" lipoprotein		Recession of childhood and	
concentrations	+10	infectious disease over past	
Having average lipoprotein		century in Western countries	+15
concentrations	0	Life insurance Impairment	
In 25th percentile of		Study	
population having		Rheumatic heart disease,	
elevated lipoproteins	−7	evidenced by:	
In 5th percentile of		Heart murmur	−11
population having		Heart murmur +	
highest elevation of		tonsillitis	−18
lipoproteins	−15	Heart murmur +	
Diabetes		streptococcal infection	−13
Uncontrolled, before insulin,		Rapid pulse	−3.5
1900	−35	Phlebitis	−3.5
Controlled with insulin		Varicose veins	−0.2
1920 Joslin Clinic record	−20	Epilepsy	−20.0
1940 Joslin Clinic record	−15	Skull fracture	−2.9
1950 Joslin Clinic record	−10	Tuberculosis	−1.8
		Nephrectomy	−2.0
		Trace of albumin in urine	−5.0
		Moderate albumin in urine	−13.5

From Jones, 1956 with permission.

as indicator of social status, leave the aged feeling powerless against the ravages of time. Accumulated stressors can invoke this sense of helpless peril and heightened vulnerability to physical and mental disease even among the normal, well elderly.

LIFE EXPECTANCY

In 1900 the life expectancy of the newborn was 47 years, but by 1950 the rate had increased to 68 years, Today the rate is 70 and 77 years for men and women respectively. Today there are more than 23,000 Americans over 100 years old while worldwide there are almost 200,000 centenarians.

Table 3-1 shows the effects of various factors on life expectancy. Examination of the environmental and physiological factors that influence life span reveals that marriage and life in rural versus urban settings may increase life expectancy by 5 years, while smoking 2 packs of cigarettes per day may reduce it by 12 years. Heredity, familial constitution, obesity, and the life-threatening effects of disease as well, are apparent in the number of years by which life may be extended or shortened.

SUMMARY

Chapter Three has examined the findings of the Duke Longitudinal Study of Normal Aging as an example of the many diverse areas of human functioning that reflect the application of adaptive and compensatory mechanisms throughout the life span. Physically, socially, and psychologically the older adult is demonstrating the ability to cope successfully. The findings also show us that senescence need not mean decline or debilitation. Certainly many physical, social or psychological processes were found to be either slowed or less reactive but an equal number were found to be stereotypical and therefore easily rejected. The relationship of health and disease states to aging were examined as factors that operate in an interdependent matrix to influence overall health practices, high-risk conditions, life expectancy, and causes of death in the older adult.

REFERENCES

Birren, J., Butler, R., Greenhouse, S., et al. (1963). *Human aging: A biological and behavioral study*. (Publication No. (HSM) 71-9051). Washington, D.C.: U.S. Government Printing Office.

Goldman, R. (1979). Aging changes in structure and function. In D. Carnevali & M. Patrick (Eds.), *Nursing management for the elderly* (pp. 53–80). Philadelphia: J.B. Lippincott.

Jones, H. A. (1956). Special consideration of the aging process. In J. Lawrence & C. Tobias (Eds.), *Advances in biological and medical physics*. (Vol. 4). New York: Academic Press.

Kalish, R. (1975). *Late adulthood: Perspectives on human development*. Monterey, CA: Brooks/Cole.

Kart, C., Metress, E., & Metress, J. (1978). *Aging and health: Biologic and social perspectives*. Menlo Park, CA: Addison Wesley.

Kimmel, D. (1980). *Adulthood and aging*. New York: Wiley and Sons.

Palmore, E. (Ed.). (1970). *Normal aging*. Durham, ND: Duke University Press.

Selye, H. (1970). Stress and aging. *Journal of the American Geriatrics Society, 18*(9), 599–690.

U.S. Department of Health, Education and Welfare. (1972). *Age patterns in medical care, illness, and disability, United States, 1968-1969*. (National Health Survey, Series 10, No. 70, National Center for Health Statistics). Washington, D.C.: U.S. Government Printing Office.

U.S. Department of Health, Education and Welfare. (1978). *Health/United States*. (Publication No. (PHS) 78-1232, Public Health Service, National Center for Health Statistics). Washington, D.C.: U.S. Government Printing Office.

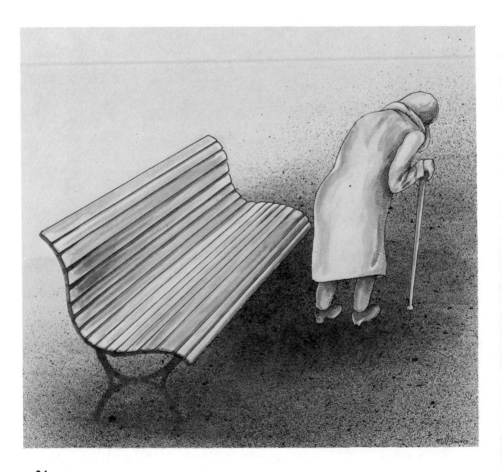

Chapter 4

Biological Change: A Review for the Psychiatric Nurse

Biological changes with age are defined as alterations in the body's structure, function, and response to illness. This has led to the formulation of some general principles.

1. Identification of a single dysfunction is unlikely since multiple dysfunctional conditions may be superimposed one upon the other.
2. Warning signals such as pain and temperature change may be absent or go unrecognized due to symptoms of prior illness or mental confusion.
3. Predisposing degenerative changes increase susceptability to infection.
4. Alterations in normal circulation and the immune system weaken resistance to infection.
5. The incidence of subclinical dietary deficiencies must be carefully considered.
6. The likelihood of mental manifestations of physical problems is great.
7. Though unchanged during a resting state, there is a measurable decline in functional reserve capacity during periods of exercise or stressful episodes.
8. The age at which disease is diagnosed can be related to the extent of pathophysiological change.
9. Sex related differences in aging are fewer in middle age than in senescence.
10. Sex related differences in disease may become more or less distinct with age.

11. Changes in one organ, organ system, or the entire body, may be premature or delayed in relation to chronological age.
12. The rate and degree of aging may vary considerably between systems.

GENERAL CHARACTERISTICS

As the body ages the more apparent changes include such common physical characteristics as graying and loss of hair, decrease in height, slower central nervous system functioning that is manifested in slower physical movement and reactivity, loss of teeth, wrinkling of skin, and impaired vision and hearing. Less apparant changes include fluctuations in the pH level of the blood, less connective tissue, reduction in the number of normal cells and cellular elements in vital organs, increased body fat, less air expired by the lungs, less oxygen utilization, less blood pumped during resting states, and a decrease in work capacity (in men a decline of 30 percent between ages 30–70 and 60 percent between ages 35–80). (Carotenuto & Bullock, 1980; Goldman, 1979).

A gradual, age-induced loss of cells has been demonstrated between older and younger organisms by measured differences in organ weight, cellular count and composition, and intracellular water. A decrease in total number of cells may reach 30 percent between youth and old age. Cellular mass has been found to decrease somewhat less, but this decrease may be obscured by increased body fat. The decrease in metabolic activity parallels that for intracellular water, while extracellular water and plasma volume tend to remain constant (Jarvik & Perl, 1981; Korenchevsky, 1961; Rockstein, Chesky & Sussman, 1977).

CHANGES IN ORGAN SYSTEMS

Cardiovascular System

For individuals over age 50 cardiovascular disease ranks as the greatest threat to life, and for those over 65 it accounts for 72 percent of all deaths. Normal age-related changes in the heart include structural and functional alterations (Rodstein, 1979). Cardiac size tends to remain relatively unchanged or even slightly decreased but increases in size have been associated with compensatory changes resulting from impaired coronary artery disease. Heart function may remain relatively constant because of this organ's ability to compensate for damage sustained by component parts.

Myocardial hypertrophy is commonly observed in the aged. In persons over age 80 the left ventricular wall may be 25 percent thicker than those age

30. There is a loss of postmitotic cardiac cells and replacement by collagen and fibrous tissue. Endocardial and valvular thickening due to collagen deposits create the appearance of white patches throughout. A thickening of myocardium is fairly common, but where disease is present the number of cells and muscle fibers are decreased and replaced by fat. Fat deposits also accumulate around the great vessels and pericardium. Lipofuscin deposition may result in a "brown heart." Myocardial changes cause a reduced stroke volume, with a decline in cardiac output and a resultant limitation in capacity for physical work. Myocardial cells also show a decreased ability to utilize oxygen.

Cardiac valves thicken and become rigid, predisposing themselves to calcification of valve cusps. Degeneration of valve cusps causes nonsignificant murmurs which have been revealed by phonocardiographic studies to be present in 60 percent or more of older individuals. More severe change is observed in the aortic valve and less severe change in the mitral valve. Within the aorta intimal hyperplasia and loss of media elasticity result in the aorta becoming dilated and unfolded. Within the coronary artery hyperplasia and fibrosis of media bring about changes so that what was formally a normal amount of physical activity or exercise for the elderly now raises heart rate and blood pressure considerably higher than desired.

Changes in the cardiac conduction system include decreased numbers of viable pacing cells, increased fibrous tissue and decreased muscle fibers. These changes result in decreased intrinsic heart rate (from 100/min to 60–80/min), possibly increased vagal tone, and lowered P, QRS and T wave amplitude on ECG examination. Lengthening of the P-R, QRS and Q-T intervals has also been found. Conduction velocity decreases except in the atrioventricular node.

Functional changes include a decrease in cardiac reserve. Capacity for cardiac response to stress, in the form of increased pulse rate, stroke volume, and cardiac output, is impaired. Cardiac output falls from five liters each minute in the 20 year old to three and a half liters each minute in the 75 year old. This decrease (0.7 percent each year after 20) is possibly due to reduced metabolic demand. There is a decrease also in stroke volume and in blood flow through coronary arteries. A decrease in blood flow of approximately 35 percent has been demonstrated from age 20 to age 60.

Vessel inelasticity, loss of cell integrity and decrease in cardiac output and stroke volume combine to produce hypoxia in organ tissue. Under ordinary conditions the normal aged heart is able to provide adequate output because of progressive decriments in metabolic rate and body atrophy. The progressive loss of stress-response capacity, however, may predispose individuals to congestive heart failure, arrhythmias, acute coronary insufficiency or myocardial necrosis.

Common pathological changes in the aged heart include:

- Cardiomegaly or hypertrophy due to long-standing congestive heart disease
- Arteriosclerotic or atherosclerotic changes in coronary arteries
- Rheumatic heart disease (mitral and aortic stenosis) in a population denied the advantages of antibiotic treatment
- Areas of scar tissue evident in myocardium due to "silent"or symptomatic myocardial infarction

Vascular changes with aging include alterations in the aorta, arteries, capillaries and veins. The aorta exhibits decreased elasticity, increased calibre, and stiffness of walls. It becomes arteriosclerotic with fibrotic changes, increased collagen and associated vascular smooth muscle loss. There is an increase in systolic blood pressure and a slighter increase in diastolic pressure. Normal blood pressure in the aged may be read at 180 mm Hg systolic and up to 110 mm Hg diastolic. Increased tortuosity is present in the aorta as well as in other arteries and arterioles. There is a loss of elastic tissue and smooth muscle. Increased mineralization (calcium), collagen deposits, and atheroma (plaques) formation as in atherosclerosis is fairly common. A decrease in vascular lumen diameter is also noted. Thickening and stiffness of basement membrane, which impairs diffusion, is found in capillaries and veins, but is not as pronounced as that found in arteries.

Functional vascular changes include a loss of resiliency leading to increases in total peripheral resistance. Losses in capillary permeability lead to slower diffusion of oxygen, nutrients and waste products throughout the vascular system. Perfusion to vital organs (heart, kidneys, brain, liver) is diminished, and baroreceptor reflexes become sluggish, predisposing to positional hypotension.

Genitourinary System

The size of the kidney decreases from young adulthood to senescence, with an approximate 30 percent loss in weight, most of which is parenchymal tissue. The number of nephrons decreases by about 30–50 percent, and those remaining are smaller in size and some are abnormal. Change begins in the areas around the capillary, with the formation of arteriovenous shunts. Hyaline deposits appear in the glomeruli and the color of the kidney darkens due to lipofuscin deposits. Vascular changes in the kidney from arteriosclerosis result in a decreased renal blood flow. Arteries become tortuous, increasing diffusion distance, and interstitial connective tissue is increased.

Functional changes include a glomerular filtration rate (GFR) that is reduced by approximately 46 percent (Sharpiro, Porush, & Kahn, 1978). Decreased membrane permeability reduces functional capacity of glomeruli and the tubular system, leading to impaired excretory and reabsorbtive capacities. Renal metabolic function is impaired and the ability to concentrate urine is lessened (at age 80 approximately 70 percent of that at age 30). No net fluid or electrolyte change is observed, but the kidney takes more time to compensate for stressors, and this ability can be overwhelmed, leading to kidney failure. Response to antidiuretic hormone is lessened, as are levels of plasma renin and aldosterone. The ability to clear urea is lessened and this is evident in increased blood urea nitrogen (BUN) levels. Glucose clearance is diminished as well. The higher incidence of nocturia in the aged may be due to better renal perfusion in a supine position as well as decreased concentration ability of the kidney (Rowe, 1976).

Pathological changes in the kidney predispose the aged to genitourinary infections, the more common of which are pyelonephritis (usually ascending from a bladder infection) and glomerulonephritis. Nephrotic syndrome, diabetic vascular changes and hypertensive renal disease, though less common, may all produce severe complications unless progressive deterioration is prevented by prompt and adequate treatment (Brocklehurst, 1979).

The consequences of age-related reduction in renal function, particularly in regard to renal excretion of drugs, has been a matter of some concern. According to Goldman (1979) 50 percent residual function is adequate when we recall that renal patients are well managed with functions as low as 5 or 10 percent of normal. Because of diminished muscle mass less creatinine is produced, with the result that serum creatinine fails to rise in proportion to the fall in renal function. As a consequence, when dosage is critical creatinine clearance rather than serum creatinine alone must be the criterion for judging renal function.

Though infection poses a threat, chronic urinary tract infections in old age are a relatively benign condition, with considerably higher incidence among institutionalized patients. It must also be pointed out that a third of patients age 65 and older have glomerular and tubular function no different than that of younger people and two-thirds exhibit normal glomerular function.

Age-related changes in the male reproductive system include hypertrophy of the prostate gland, softening and reduced size of the testicles, reduced production of sperm (although abundant spermatozoa may be found even in advanced age), thickening of the seminiferous tubules with a reduction in diameter, and reduction in blood flow to the penis. Although it gradually declines, testosterone production continues well into old age.

Age-related changes in the female reproductive system are characterized by reduction in estrogen production with the onset of menopause. The uterus and ovaries become smaller. There is some vulva atrophy, and atrophy of the vaginal mucosa and glands. The vaginal lining becomes thin and pale. There is a narrowing and shortening of the vagina, with a decrease in elasticity, size of vaginal opening, and vaginal lubrication. Estrogen deficiency alters the pH of the vaginal environment, increasing the likelyhood of dyspereunia and vaginitis. This deficiency also reduces the glandular tissue of the breast.

Hematopoietic System

There is remarkably little change in the hematopoietic system with age. Changes in circulating blood volume, erythrocyte count, and hemoglobin level of normal, well elderly persons living at home and remaining socially active are only minimal. Those of institutionalized persons show a slight decrease in value. Good health maintenance has been shown by some studies to influence erythrocyte count and hemoglobin level (Maekawa, 1976; Shapleigh, Mayes, & Moore, 1952). Subjects who had regular physical examinations and followed recommended health regimens had higher levels of both erythrocyte and hemoglobin, in contrast to those who did not.

Only subtle change is found in the red blood cells, and the number and distribution of leukocytes remains unchanged. Anemia is common in advanced age and is usually caused by iron deficiency. The erythrocyte sedimentation rate may be accelerated even in the absence of disease, but this may be more attributable to changes in plasma proteins, particularly fibrinogen.

Changes due to aging in hematopoietic cells in bone marrow are minimal, but fatty marrow gradually replaces active hematopoietic marrow. Plasma iron, total iron binding capacity, and ferritin show slight decline with age.

Respiratory System

Several age-related changes take place in the respiratory system that alter the mechanical aspects of respiration as well as pulmonary diffusion and capacity (Malasanos, Barkauskas, Moss, & Stollenberg-Allen, 1981; Murray & Zentner, 1979). There is greater rigidity of the airways and tissues with age. Decreased elasticity of costal cartilage and progressive kyphosis increase the rigidity of the chest wall. Respiratory muscle weakness decreases functional reserve capacity.

Functional residual capacity increases with age (50 percent from the third to the ninth decade) resulting in only partial inflation of the lungs at rest. Despite this there is no significant change in total lung capacity. Sclerosis of the bronchi and supporting tissues, and degeneration of bronchial epithelium decrease vital capacity and reduce forced expiratory volume (FEV).

Coalescence of the alveoli result in the diaphragm and abdominal wall musculature becoming increasingly important in effecting ventilation. Diffusion capacity is diminished. With matched pulmonary blood flow rates, the 80 year old actually receives only one third the oxygen into the cardiovascular system as the 20 year old, and hence must breathe longer and harder. Uniformity of ventilation with quiet breathing is lessened, and the maximal amount of oxygen utilized under stress is decreased 50 percent by age 80.

Degeneration of mucosal glands lessens efficiency of the pulmonary cleansing mechanism. Rigidity of the thoracic wall and lessened strength of expiratory muscles diminish the propulsive efficiency of the cough. Lessened cough efficiency, decreased ciliary activity in the bronchial lining, and greater dead space all increase the likelihood of mechanical and infectious complications following surgery or enforced bed rest.

Integumentary System

Normal changes in the integumentary system with age are evident in skin, hair and related somatic functions (Tindall, 1978). The skin becomes thin, dry, inelastic and wrinkled with hanging folds. It assumes a paler, more fragile coloration with an increase in discoloration and pigmentation. Normal epidermal overgrowth appears as raised pale, brown, or black warts (hyperkeratoses). Hair growth diminishes over the entire body. Nail growth is slower. Atrophy of the epidermis, sweat glands and hair follicles causes a loss of existing hair, particularly in the scalp. Fewer melanocytes cause less pigment granules and result in a graying of hair color.

The degeneration of collagen and elastin result in senile purpura. A thickening of blood vessels results in cherry angiomata (de Morgan spots). Somatic mutations as well are present in the form of atrophic or deformed nails. A loss of subcutaneous fat causes much of the wrinkling of skin and a diminished tolerance for heat and cold. This fat loss also increases vulnerability to heat exhaustion because of changes in perspiration capacity and atrophied sweat glands. A more serious complication of lessened subcutaneous fat is a loss of body padding and subsequent predisposition to decubitous ulcers. Immobilization need not be extensive to cause decubiti. Studies have demonstrated that one in three pressure sores developes within the first week of institutionlization, and two in three develop within the first two weeks. The sensitivity of the skin is obvious here and in a predisposition to physiological and biochemical responsivity to environment. The ravages of overexposure to sunshine or dermatologic agents in soaps, non-prescription ointments and toxic chemicals have been widely reported. A need for greater healing time and a gradual loss of healing capacity can cause even minor trauma to result in major problems.

Gastrointestinal System

Changes in the gastrointestinal system with age begin with the digestive process (Malasanos et al., 1981). Dentition and mastication of food are both affected by aging. Approximately 50 percent of all Americans have lost a majority of teeth by age 65 and almost 75 percent are totally edentulous by age 75. Much of this loss is attributable to individual and professional neglect, the costs involved in dental health, or deficits in early childhood dental health education. Dental carries, a major source of tooth loss prior to age 35, is replaced after age 40 by pyorrhea. In either case improper chewing of food for digestion can increase the likelihood of indigestion and reinforce a preference for nutritionally inadequate soft foods.

Some atrophy of the mucosa, intestinal glands, and the muscularis is associated with aging. The volume of saliva produced diminishes. There is a decrease in salivary ptylin and with it a decrease in starch digestion. Decline in production of hydrochloric acid pepsin, and pancreatic enzymes (amylase, lipase, trypsin) may account for anorexia and indigestion with age. Dysphagia is a common problem and may be due to either structural changes within the esophagus, lessened esophageal motility, or an increase in nonpropulsive contractions. Difficulty in swallowing when in a supine position and an increased incidence of aspiration have been reported. The incidence of hiatal hernia is also common, present in 70 percent of individuals over age 70.

While few other changes are associated with the small intestine because of organic cellular renewal well into advanced age, changes in absorption are fairly common. The villa of the mucosa of the small bowel become shorter and broader, diminishing the amount of absorption surface. Studies of glucose absorption have been difficult to interpret because of fluctuations in glucose–insulin relationship, but findings suggest a decrease in the absorption rate of fats, calcium, and vitamins B^1 and B^{12}.

Within the pancreas, alveolar degeneration and duct obstruction have been reported, but the evidence regarding proteolytic enzyme activity has been inconclusive. Changes in the gallbladder have been limited to the common presence of calculi and the consequences of cholecystic infection, rather than to aging itself. A known decrease in size of the liver has been evident for some time, decreasing from approximately 1929 gm in the fourth decade to 1000 gm in the tenth, with the greatest decline after the sixth decade. Bilirubin clearance is unaffected, and no significant difference between young and old has been found for total serum bilirubin, SGOT, and SGPT valves. Change in liver cells (loss of mitochondria, lipofuscin accumulation, endoplasmic reticulum change), enzyme function, storage capacity and hepatic blood flow are fairly slight and require additional critical evaluation. Decreases reported in the liver's synthetic function (protein synthesis) and microsomal oxidase activity (drug and steroid metabolism) are slight and unaccompanied by decline in general liver function. To date there is little real evidence, in the absence of specific pathophysiological change, of disturbance in liver function.

Endocrine System

The literature on endocrine change in aging is inconclusive in many respects. Studies conducted on rats and other laboratory animals have not correlated well with age-related changes in human physiology. Several researchers have speculated that the changes in endocrine function may be related to the involution of the endocrine system and caused by a biological clock or by autoimmunity (Andres & Tobin, 1972; Everitt & Huang, 1980; Matsuyama & Jarvik, 1980). At this time there is a paucity of data available on systemic endocrine alteration with age. The integrative nature of the endocrine system is such that imbalance within the renal system (reduced GFR), when combined with impaired respiratory function (less diffusion capacity), results in less acid–base balance and greater vulnerability to fluctuations in blood pH. Despite sparse and often conflicting findings some changes appear to be taking place with age that affect most other systems of the body.

The pituitary gland appears to maintain normal functional levels as master gland and regulator of other glands, despite reports of a decrease in some cell types and in pituitary activity with age. Specific hormones differ somewhat from their former levels but appear to be little affected by age. A reported decrease in growth hormone (somatotropin) may be more a function of differences between the obese and non-obese subjects studied, or a response to insulin provocation. Thyroid stimulating hormone (thyrotropin) seems to be changed little if at all. ACTH (corticotropin) appears to remain unchanged in normal functions, but circadian rhythms may be altered. A complex interrelationship exists between hormones secreted by the hypothalamus, anterior pituitary and gonads. Though the exact role of the hypothalamic–pituitary axis in the control of reproduction is not fully understood, morphological change has been observed. The anterior lobe of the pituitary has exhibited significant histological change in postmenopausal women, with greatest change found in gonadotrophin-secreting basophil cells. No change has been found in the hypothalams.

A further relationship between hypothalamic–pituitary interaction is of interest because of potential implications to endocrine change with aging; neurotransmitter catecholamines are thought to participate in the regulation of hypothalamic hormones. Increasing research attention is being paid to the hypothalamic–pituitary complex, and its interacting CNS, hypothalamus, and anterior pituitary components, because of speculation that decreased pituitary function and decreased hypothalamic stimulating hormones (neurotransmitters) may both be related to mental changes such as confusion and depression.

Change in the thyroid is characterized by a decreased basal metabolic rate commensurate with age and decline in physical activity. Less radioiodine accumulation in the thyroid has been reported (Everitt & Huang, 1980).

Plasma thyroxine (T_4), both protein-bound and free, appears to be unaffected by age. Plasma triiodothyronine (T_3), however, has been shown to decrease 25–40 percent after the sixth decade. Normal plasma T_4 concentration, and a reduction in radioiodine uptake by the thyroid, suggest that the rates of destruction and replacement of the hormone are slowed in proportion to uptake rates of younger adults. Thyroid disease is fairly common in the elderly. Hypo- and hyperthyroidism may result in atypical, nonspecific symptoms; as many as five years may be required to correctly diagnose the condition. Since many of the symptoms are behavioral rather than physical, a diagnostic problem of major proportions resulted. The classic clinical picture of thyroid disease in the elderly has too frequently been diagnosed as "dementia" rather than endocrine disorder, with resulting complications that seriously jeopardize the overall wellbeing of the patient (Jarvik & Perl, 1981). This syndrome is discussed in Chapter 6.

The major change in the parathyroid gland is in structure (a significant increase in number of oxyphilic cells), while function is believed to be maintained unimpaired throughout life. Changes in other glands may influence its activity levels slightly. An increase in parathyroid hormone (PTH) has been associated with osteoporosis, while heightened physiological sensitivity to this disorder has resulted from postmenopausal decrease in estrogen production. Overproduction of PTH is one cause of hypercalcemia, a disorder of relatively high incidence in the elderly and one that exhibits neuropsychiatric symptoms.

Changes in the pancreas suggest that insulin production may be reduced or delayed due to reduced beta cell response to hyperglycemia. A constant rate of decrease in glucose tolerance has been demonstrated frequently. Elevated serum glucose levels suggest that over half of all elderly persons are diabetic, and therefore glucose tolerance tests have limited use in the diagnosis of diabetes in the elderly (Andres & Tobin, 1972). While only 5 percent of individuals under age 40 will have blood glucose levels over 165 mg/dl, two hours after an oral glucose load of 1.75 mg/kg, 35 percent of those over age 70 will have higher levels. Furthermore, many of the elderly with reduced glucose tolerance appear to be in good health and unlikely to develop overt diabetes. Glucose intolerance is also known to be associated with stress. In fact, present standard values must be revised to reflect age-related increases in glucose intolerance, rather than be used to imply that inadequate insulin production exists. Several indicators suggest that insulin production remains normal with aging but loses efficacy. Tissue sensitivity to insulin, and the efficiency of insulin in controlling glucose levels, have both been found to decrease with age. The incidence of diabetes mellitus in advanced age is quite common, and extensive research on glucose intolerance is presently underway (Andres & Tobin, 1972, 1977).

Few histological changes in the adrenals have been reported in the elderly. These glands appear able to maintain their ability to respond to

ACTH by increasing levels of cortisol. Peripheral elimination of cortisol is reduced with age, but this may be due to impairment of the liver or kidneys. Contradictory findings for reduced adrenal response to corticotropin stimulation have also been reported, which may be significant to future research on stress–response capabilities.

Musculoskeletal System

Changes in the musculature of the body are evident in a progressive decline in muscle mass, atrophy of some muscle groups, and a loss of muscle strength. The replacement of contractile fibers with connective tissue adds to a loss of muscle strength and endurance. A decrease in the number of muscle cells with age is significant, linear, and in excess of loss of essential neural components. Losses in muscle strength contribute to stiff body movements, irregular gait, and vulnerability to injury.

Muscle tissue becomes the site of lipofuscin deposition, resulting in diminished density of capillaries in each motor unit. There is a significant reduction in the capacity of some enzyme systems that affect muscles, but oxygen utilization in each unit of tissue remains essentially unchanged.

Body musculature experiences a prolongation about 13 percent of contraction time, latency period, and relaxation period. A decrease is seen in the maximum rate of tension development. Since functional loss in one system will inevitably influence functional capacity in another, normal muscle function may be impaired by decreased cardiac output. The decrease in motor function may be compounded by other factors such as poor motivation, malnutrition, deconditioning, endocrine changes, or normal involutional processes.

Changes in joints are characterized by major deterioration of cartilage, a process that can begin as early as the third decade. Such changes are often associated with cumulative trauma, and result in a form of degenerative arthritis accompanied by pain, crepitation, and limitation of movement. Osteoarthritic changes in joints are highly characteristic of aging and easily verified by x-ray. Estimation of age by examination of proliferative change in the cervical spine has been claimed by roentgenologists to be relatively easy due to characteristic profusion and lipping of the vertibrae, and development of bony overgrowths.

There is a loss of ligament and cartilage resilience and elasticity. Degeneration, erosion, and calcification takes place in both cartilage and ligaments. Functional changes include a decline in fine movement precision, a decline in rapid alternating movement, irregularity in timing and smooth flow from one action to another, and a lessening of confidence in motor movement. The body posture becomes slightly stooped and some height is generally lost, attributable in part to a narrowing of joint spaces, particularly of the intervertebral disks.

Changes in bone begin prior to age 40 with a shift from an increase in bone mass to a progressive decrease. In long and flat bones a gradual reabsorption of the interior surface and a slower accretion of new bone on exterior surfaces occurs, so that these bones are enlarged outside and hollowed within. Vertebral end plates become thinned, and the skull slightly enlarged. Trabeculae are lost resulting in weaker bone, more vulnerable to fracture. Atrophy of bone (osteoporosis and osteomalacia) may be attributed to immobility, failure to absorb calcium, excessive calcium loss from the bowel or kidney, or endocrine disorders. Remodeling of bone increases with age within the haversian system. Bones become more porous, mineralization decreases, the number of blocked Haversian canals increases, and greater numbers of osteocytes die. The decline in bone mass is estimated to be from 5–10 percent each decade.

Osteoporosis is less a pathological finding than the absence of normal findings. The first indication of osteoporosis may be the presence of kyphosis, with characteristic painful changes in the vertebral column. With its onset, the entire skeleton experiences a loss of cortical thickness, increased porosity in normal bone, and a thinning of cancellous bone. Bone loss in females is estimated to be approximately 25 percent, and in males 12 percent. Given the smaller female frame a loss of this magnitude helps explain the greater number of fractures in women. Senile osteoporosis is the most common metabolic bone disorder in this country, and provides predisposition to 75 percent of all upper femur fractures.

Nervous System

Both structural and functional changes take place in the nervous system with age. Macroscopic changes are evident in a reduction in brain weight and size. Atrophy of the brain results in a separation of the surface of the brain from the skull, and an enlargement of ventricles. A general rule of thumb applies to the reduction in brainweight—a 5 percent loss by age 70, 10 percent by age 80, and 20 percent by age 90. Decreases in volume are also apparent in brain mass, with a decline of approximately 200 cc in men from age 20 to age 80, and a corresponding increase in extracerebral space of approximately 200 cc. There is also a widening and deepening of the sulci, a narrowing of gyri, and enlargement of ventricles (Drachman, 1980).

Circulation and oxygen utilization in the brain have been extensively studied. Cerebral blood flow has been shown to decrease some 20 percent by age 80. Goldman (1979) reported that from the second to eighth decades mean arterial pressure remained at 90–110 mm Hg, but cerebral blood flow declines from 79 ml/min to 46 ml/min for each 100 gm of brain tissue. The rate of cerebral oxygen consumption also decreased, from 3.6 ml O_2/min to 27 ml O_2/min for each 100 gm brain tissue.

The rate of cell loss varies, but overall loss may be as much as 45 percent in some cortical areas and 25 percent in the cerebellum. Some investigators have found significant losses in the superior frontal gyrus and marked changes in pyramidal cells of the cerebral cortex.

Adams (1980) has identified several factors in the process of neuronal degeneration that are characteristic of aging. Synaptic and dendritic surfaces of neurons showed degeneration of apical shafts, and a progressive loss of horizontally oriented dendritic systems. Axons became thinner and myelin sheaths were found to thicken as axons diminished in size. Axosomatic and axodendritic synapses were reduced in number. Synthetic enzymes were also found to decline in relation to neuronal changes. Those that produced catecholamines were reduced, while monoamine oxidase was shown to increase.

Lipofuscin accumulation has been a known concomitant of aging cells for over a century. It manifests itself in the nervous system in the form of fine granules that collect in the cytoplasm of neurons, between the nucleus and apical dendrite. Its pigment, commonly stained brown, occurs in cells throughout the body, and is consequently referred to as the "wear and tear" pigment. Accumulation is greatest in storage vacuoles, and this accumulation has a high quantitative correlation with aging. Despite the degree of research interest its ubiquity has generated, the effect of its presence on cell function is still unknown.

Neurofibrillary tangles proliferate into compact parallel bundles that displace the neuronal nucleus as they fill out the cytoplasmic space. It is theorized (Adams, 1980; Drachman, 1980) that neurofibrillary tangles indicate an abnormality of protein metabolism. Their proliferation results in eventual neuronal death. Their more common sites (in the absence of disease) are the hippocampus and temporal and frontal lobes of the cortex. Curiously, they are not evident in sensory neurons of the dorsal-root ganglia, spinal cord, or brainstem.

Granulovacuolar degeneration consists of the formation of dense basophilic granules surrounded by vacuoles. These granules are more evident in cases where senile plaques and fibrillary changes are present, and although a prominent feature of senile dementia and Alzheimer's disease, it is also found in normal aging brains. Senile plaques vary in size and shape, and consist of granular, filamentous debris that is localized mainly in the cerebral cortex.

Findings regarding changes in the autonomic nervous system have been inconclusive. Everitt and Huang (1980) have stated that the significance of the autonomic system in aging has not been adequately or systematically studied. Current knowledge of the relationship of autonomic failure to normal aging is limited to speculation. Maximal degenerative change has been seen in the limbic area of patients with Alzheimer's disease, but no neuron loss has been associated with age-related change in the hypothalamus of human subjects.

Compensation to neurological aging and neurological disease seems to be quite possible. Individuals who had been functioning normaly have been found upon autopsy to show extensive disease of neural structures, while individuals with senile dementia have retained considerable intellectual function. The question of whether diseases such as senile dementia, so closely linked to degenerative central nervous system change, are manifestations of aging or of disease has not been resolved. There is not sufficient evidence that accumulations of lipofuscin, plaque formation, or neurofibrillary proliferation are causative, or even related, to neuronal loss.

REFERENCES

Adams, R. (1980). The morphological aspects of aging in the human nervous system. In J. Birren & R. Sloane (Eds.), *Handbook of mental health and aging* (pp. 149–160). Englewood Cliffs, NJ: Prentice-Hall. 149–160.

Andres, R., & Tobin, J. (1972). Aging, carbohydrate metabolism and diabetes. *Proceedings of the Ninth International Congress of Gerontology*, 1, (pp. 276–280).

Andres, R. & Tobin, J. (1977). Endocrine systems. In C. Finch & L. Hayflick (Eds.), *Handbook of the biology of aging* (pp. 357–378). New York: Van Nostrand Reinhold Co.

Brocklehurst, J. (1979). The urinary tract. In I. Rossman (Ed.), *Clinical geriatrics*. (2nd ed.) (pp. 317–330). Philadelphia: Lippincott Co.

Carotenuto, R. & Bullock, J. (1980). *Physical assessment of the gerontologic client*. Philadelphia: F. A. Davis.

Drachman, D. (1980). An approach to the neurology of aging. In J. Birren & R. Sloane (Eds.), *Handbook of mental health and aging* (pp. 501–519). Englewood Cliffs, NJ: Prentice-Hall.

Everitt, A. and Huang, C. (1980). The hypothalamus, neuroendocrine and autonomic nervous systems in aging. In J. Birren & R. Sloane (Eds.), *Handbook of mental health and aging* (pp. 100–133). Englewood Cliffs, NJ: Prentice-Hall.

Goldman, R. (1979). Aging changes in structure and function. In D. Carnevali & M. Patrick (Eds.), *Nursing management for the elderly*. Philadelphia: Lippincott Co.

Jarvik, L. & Perl, M. (1981). Overview of physiologic dysfunctions related to psychiatric problems in the elderly. In A. Levensen & R. Hall (Eds.), *Neuropsychiatric manifestations of physical disease in the elderly*. (Vol. 14 Aging Series) (pp. 1–15). New York: Raven Press.

Korenchevsky, V. (1961). *Physiological and pathological aging*. New York: Hafner Publishing Co.

Libow, L. (1963). Medical investigation of the processes of aging. In J. Birren, R. Butler, S. Greenhouse et al. (Eds.), *Human aging: A Biological and behavioral study*. Publication No. (HSM) 71-9051 (p. 37). Washington, DC: U.S. Government Printing Office.

Maekawa, T. (1976). Hematologic diseases. In F. Sternberg (Ed.), *Cowdry's the care of the geriatric patient* (pp. 152–166). St. Louis: C. V. Mosby Co.

Malasanos, L., Barkauskas, V., Moss, M. & Stollenberg-Allen, K. (1981). *Health assessment*. St. Louis: C. V. Mosby.
Matsuyama, S. & Jarvik, L. (1980). Genetic and mental functioning in senescence. In J. Birren & R. Sloane (Eds.), *Handbook of mental health and aging* (pp. 134–148). Englewood Cliffs, NJ: Prentice-Hall.
Murray, R. & Zentner, J. (1979). *Nursing assessment and health promotion through the life span* (2nd ed.). Englewood Cliffs, NJ: Prentice-Hall.
Rockstein, M., Chesky, J., & Sussman, M. (1979). Comparative biology and evolution of aging. In C. Finch and L. Hayflick (Eds.), *Handbook of the biology of aging* (pp. 3–34). New York: Van Nostrand Reinhold Co.
Rodstein, M. (1979). Heart disease in the aged. In I. Rossman (Ed.), *Clinical geriatrics* (2nd ed.) (pp. 181–203). Philadelphia: Lippincott Co.
Rowe, J. (1976). The effect of age on creatinine clearance in men: A cross sectional and longitudinal study. *Journal of Gerontology, 31,* 155–163.
Shapiro, W., Porush, J., & Kahn, A. (1978). Medical renal diseases in the aged. In W. Reichel (Ed.), *Clinical aspects of aging* (pp. 199–212). Baltimore: Williams and Wilkins Co.
Shapleigh, J., Mayes, S., & Moore, C. (1952). Hematologic values in the aged. *Journal of Gerontology, 7,* 207–219.
Tindall, J. (1978). Geriatric dermatology. In W. Reichel (Ed.), *Clinical Aspects of Aging* (pp. 331–356). Baltimore: Williams and Wilkins Co.

SUGGESTED READINGS

Conconi, F., Manenti, F., & Benatti, F.G. (1963). Behavior of some enzyme activities in plasma in normal subjects in relation to age. *Acta Vitaminologica, 17,* 33–35.
Cutler, J. (1970). Normal values for multiphasic screening blood chemistry test. In *Advances in automated analysis* (Vol. III: Technicon International Congress, 1969) (pp. 67–73). White Plains, NY: Medaid, Inc.
Davidshohn, I., & Henry, J. (Eds.) (1974). *Todd-Sanford clinical diagnosis by laboratory methods,* (ed. 15) (pp. 1376–1392). Philadelphia: W. B. Saunders Co.
Hayes, G. & Stinson, I. (1976). Erythrocyte sedimentation rate and age. *Archives of Ophthalmology, 94,* 939–940.
Talley, L. (1979). Laboratory values. In D. Carnevali & M. Patrick (Eds.), *Nursing management for the elderly* (pp. 81–110). Philadelphia: Lippincott Co.
Werner, M. (1970). Influence of sex and age on the normal range of eleven serum constituents. *Zeitschrift fur Klinische Chemie and Klinische Biochemie, 8,* 105–115.
Wilding, P., Rollason, J., & Robinson, D. (1972). Patterns of change for various biochemical constituents detected in well population screening. *Clinica Chimica Acta, 41,* 375–387.

Introduction
Assessment and Aging

Part II addresses the systematic collection and analysis of data on the health status of the aged patient. Chapter 5 examines various components of mental status assessment, including the interview, history, mental status examination, and mental status questionnaire. The interaction of age, systemic disease, altered central nervous system function, drugs, stress and nutrition, all of which may induce symptoms of apparent psychogenic etiology, are discussed in Chapter 6. Certain common recurring problems seen in the older patient are treated in Chapter 7. These include confusion (a frequent symptom of underlying physiogenic illness), depression (which commonly overlays other organic problems), and senile psychosis, all of which are examined as dysfunctional syndromes requiring differential assessment. Because of the need for reduction in false positive and false negative diagnoses, acute and chronic mental syndromes are dealt with separately in Chapter 8.

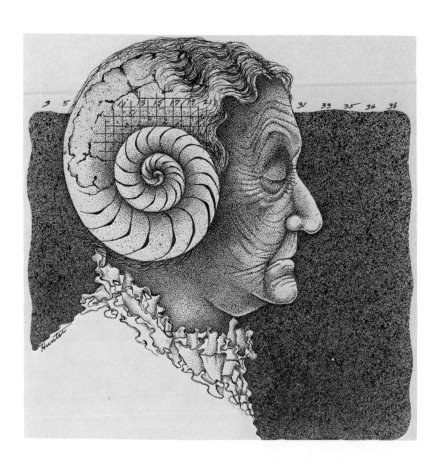

Chapter 5

Assessment of Mental Process

The intent to assess the health status of someone automatically infers an intent to intervene somehow in the life of the person being assessed, but the assessment process is only as accurate, comprehensive, or unbiased, as the person carrying it out. The assessor's astuteness, professional acumen, and willingness to look well beyond stereotypes is nowhere more essential than in assessment of the aged patient.

The psychiatric nurse who undertakes the assessment of geriatric mental health is burdened by the varied dimensions of the geriatric personality that may reflect problems as varied as accentuated premorbidity, late-onset depression, confusional episodes, or even underlying renal disease. Intermittent fluctuations in sensorium resulting from multiple physiological, pharmacological, or social causes, compound the problem.

Assessment is difficult, and assessment of mental health status of the elderly is at times tortuous. It involves the determination of whether or not the presented behavior is indicative of normal aging or psychopathology, and, if determined to be psychopathologic in nature, whether it is of functional or organic etiology. All interventions and treatment recommendations derive from assessment that is precise, that answers well-posited questions. This chapter focuses on specific issues and topics that should aid the reader in the assessment process.

THE ASSESSMENT PROCESS

Older subjects differ from the young in many ways. Neuronally transmitted impulses are slower and fewer in number. Performance aspects of intelligence and the ability to solve problems are reduced. Concentration is more difficult. The aged patient may oversimplify, concretize, and overcautiously avoid any risk of failure or threat to self-esteem.

Underreporting illness is more likely, while the ability to identify stressors is less likely. Memory is poor. Visual and auditory losses limit the ability to receive, interpret, and respond to stimuli. Neural noise confuses, distorts, and obscures interpersonal communication. Aged persons may believe that their frame of reference is so inapplicable to the situation at hand that little value is attached to communication efforts. Or, the need to communicate clearly may remain great, but the ability to clarify the problem is severely restricted. All of these factors hinder the assessment process by limiting the patient's ability to identify and accurately articulate just what is wrong, an impediment that obscures their present health status and imposes a greater-than-normal burden on the interviewer's interpersonal skills.

The assessment of mental health should be dictated by the needs of the patient, and nowhere is the need for genuine interest and empathy more essential than in assessment of the inarticulate aged. A relationship is developed between patient and provider that influences all future contacts by that patient within the health care system, so it behooves the provider to remain acutely sensitive to responses from the patient.

Because the human organism is actually many small systems linked by internal transactions, Lomax (1982) suggests that the elements of any illness process be assessed in terms of transactions between systems of bodily, personal, and social functions, as well as the integrating mechanisms between the systems. Every organism relates to its various parts as a functional whole that, in turn, relates to the natural environment and, in the case of humans, to family and society. Purposeful observations must be made by the assessor at levels of progressively increasing complexity, ranging from enzymatic and organ systems through family and sociocultural systems. The nature of geriatric mental illness must, therefore, be viewed as a final common pathway of dysfunction in one or more levels of the aggregate of linked systems that is the aged patient.

The underlying causes of mental disorder are varied, but Gurland (1980) suggests that for some purposes the effects on the elderly patient can be classified into a relatively limited range of categories. These categories constitute the final common pathways of mental disorder, and are determined by selective input from formal sources, such as the health care system, and informal sources, such as family or significant others. The range of categories is limited by several factors; the nature of the mental disorder, the repertoire of inherited or acquired behaviors, the methods currently available to detect abnormalities of behavior, and the targets of helping responses by formal and informal agents. Mental health assessment of the aged patient usually begins with an examination of each of these final common pathways.

- Cognitive impairment
- Depression

- Excessive dependence on others
- Disruptive/dangerous behavior
- Bizarre behavior
- Somatic disturbance
- Social maladjustment

The assessment of mental process requires the identification of symptoms suggesting organic damage as well as symptoms of phenomenological psychopathology. These may include:

- Depressed mood
- Phobic anxiety
- Somatic (vegetative) complaints
- Thought disorder
- Hallucinations
- Delusions
- Motor and speech retardation
- Obsessions
- Depersonalization
- Drug/alcohol abuse
- Impaired insight
- Hypochondriasis
- Apathy and withdrawal
- Impaired concentration
- Antisocial behavior
- Diminished memory, orientation, and judgement

Merely identifying the symptom is insufficient, however, since detailed fluctuations in symptomatology (i.e., diurinal variation in mood) are particularly important. In addition, premorbid personality as described by family or friends, prior episodes, length of intervals between episodes, when illness first occurs, course and response to treatment, family history, precipitating events, familial reinforcement, and the patient's physical health status are equally significant to any comprehensive assessment profile.

One of the most challenging aspects of geriatric assessment involves the differentiation of organic from functional pathology. Organic mental syndrome is discussed in detail in Chapter 8, but it should be noted here that in the absence of organic damage wide-range neuropsychological disturbances should not be present, the patient's orientation to time, place, and person should be good, response to interviewer's questions may be slowed but otherwise accurate, and no manifest speech disturbances should be present.

The major task involves what Small (1973) describes as identification of the "criterion problem," or, that clearly differentiated problem against which comparative estimations of mental health status may be made (i.e., discrete populations of schizophrenic patients without brain damage, or brain-damaged patients with schizophrenia). Although a single criterion problem may be more easily identified in younger patients, in the aged every indication suggests the presence of multiple criterion problems. This phenomenon is discussed thoroughly in Chapter 6. Consequently, what is required on the part of assessors is cognizance of the likelihood of multiple criterion problems and documentation of their common final pathway effects. To that end Small recommends use of a series of interview questions that when answered, yield substantive data.

1. What is the presenting complaint that has motivated the patient to seek or be brought for treatment? It may be the real problem or merely a masked derivative of other pathways.

2. What precipitated the complaint? The psychosocial context within which the complaint became apparent may reveal a great deal of valuable information about how the patient has reacted or not reacted to illness.

3. What are the antecedent analogues of the present complaint? Information on similar episodes will aid in understanding the psychodynamic history or illuminate the recency of the isolated event.

4. What are the meanings of the symptoms? Do they signal to the patient or family evidence of "madness" requiring institutionalization? What are the emotional responses?

5. What is the state of the ego system? Manifestations of strengthened or weakened ego functions will aid in the identification of necessary changes and the selection of appropriate interventions.

6. What shifts are necessary to restore homeostasis? Will ego be strengthened by increasing or weakening a particular defense, or can social maladjustment be corrected by therapeutic contact with people?

7. What interventions will produce the desired homeostatic shift? *Is* any intervention required? If so, should it be primarily psychotherapeutic and secondarily sociotherapeutic, or vice versa?

8. What therapeutic allies are available? Are the patient's inner resources (confidence, intelligence, awareness, etc.) available and/or what familial and social resources can be summoned?

9. What therapeutic procedural recommendations are indicated? Once specific goals are identified, how should they be prioritized? Should family conferences be conducted while medical treatment is underway?

10. What is the prognosis? Is the expectation of improvement realistic or optimistic? Is chemotherapy preferable to psychotherapy or sociotherapy? What effect will the prognosis have on the patient, staff, and family?

THE INTERVIEW

In contrast to the medical interview where most patients are actively seeking help and where cooperation is usually high, the mental assessment interview, as Feinberg (1975) reminds us, may be characterized by patient motivation that is variable at best. Many patients are present against their will, and still others have opposing forces within them that mitigate the possibility of them revealing information.

The purpose of the interview should be known to the patient with sufficient time allowed for exploration of salient details. Privacy, confidentiality, and respect for the patient's rights must be maintained. The setting should be quiet and free of interruption. Comfort and good lighting are recommended. Communication should be solely at a level the patient understands, and free of colloquialisms and medicalese. Full facial contact, body language, and change-of-topic "signals" should be used. The interviewer should be prepared to clarify whatever is not fully understood, and to summarize the major points covered. Since maximal spontaneity is desired, interviewer interventions should be limited to those that clarify and encourage further dialogue rather than those that force movement and direction. Factual data, or "the words of the song," may be far less revealing that the "musical theme" itself, so the interviewer should be attuned to both.

Elderly patients are frequently reluctant to acknowledge sensory losses, and may also deny deficits in self-care activity. The stereotype of an "old" person unwilling to devulge personal information to a "young" professional is, however, unfounded. More often than not they desire contact with the young but are justifiably concerned with being typecasted in undesirable roles, such as a "cute old granny."

Anxiety among the elderly is commonly high, particularly when awareness of failing sensory or motor skills is uppermost in their mind. They may suspect that they are "going crazy" yet be very ambivalent about any outside intervention. Feelings of helplessness at their plight, and a desire for help, may be offset by feelings of anger, even outraged betrayal, toward family members. The interviewer must focus attention on those thoughts or environmental strains that precipitate or increase anxiety. Similarly, depression is so common that the shortened attention span and reiteration of destructive, self-deprecatory statements by patients may require not only noting, but active interruption and refocusing by the interviewer. Special note must be made of any suicidal ideas or distructive behavior.

HISTORY TAKING

The history is usually elicited from the patient, relatives, and friends. Freedman, Kaplan, and Sadock (1976) stress the importance of identifying the circumstances surrounding the initial contact. The patient's perception of the present situation is especially revealing, and encouraging the patient to describe the chief complaint in terms of a topic he considers most important is strongly advised. Past negative experiences with nurses and doctors may have left the patient feeling frustrated, puzzled, and misunderstood, so it is essential that the patient be given ample opportunity to prioritize a "chief complaint," be it medical, familial, or social.

The medical history is of critical significance to the assessor of the aged patient, and must address all past illnesses and operations, their complications and outcomes, and the patient's reactions. Any drug-taking habits and past central nervous system dysfunction must be noted. The review of systems (ROS) will reveal the patient's ability to recall dates of illness, the nature of symptoms, and offer some indication of individual ability to cope with stress. Memory loss will prevent the patient from recalling all pertinent injuries or communicable diseases sustained, so he should be asked to identify only those that stand out in memory as unusual.

The patient's present orientation to mental well-being can often be illuminated by a retrospective account of past experiences and their residual effects. The past history will cover formal and informal education and training, occupational and military experience, and the development of peer relationships. Periods of psychological dysfunction, and the adjustment mechanisms employed to cope with them, will often reveal many aspects of the patient's personality—attitudes, self esteem, reactions to others, and general psychological orientation. Episodic psychiatric illness, and treatment measures used, should be identified and described.

Personal history data should include current living conditions, existing social relationships, derived values and beliefs, and in general what the individual sees as personal strengths and weaknesses. Asking the patient to describe a typical 24-hour day will shed much light on perceptions of self, reality, and position in society. The completed personal history should describe the patient's characteristic response to developmental challenges, psychological defenses, and self image. Feinberg recommends that the personal history, far from being merely a routine listing of biographical events, should attempt to answer four major questions.

1. How has the patient responded to major developmental and environmental challenges?
2. What are the main modes of dealing with psychological stress, i.e., what is the characteristic personality style?
3. How has the patient dealt historically with reality and interpersonal intimacy?
4. What is the patient's self image?

The family history is used to gather data on biological, social, and familial circumstances. Questions pertaining to the patient's ancestors and any genetic predisposition to conditions or diseases, and the causes of death of parents and grandparents, may all help in the development of a comprehensive treatment plan. A description of the patient's past and present family units should address parental attitudes and values; how the patient was reared, and how the patient parented his children. How is the patient's family described as a social system? What roles do members play? What rules shape values and communication between members? What is the socioeconomic status of the family? What alliances exist among members, and how do they affect members' needs for physical and emotional support?

The social history examines levels of competency in regard to social roles, participation in communal activities, capacity for purposeful and meaningful interaction with others, and maintenance of independent self-care activities. Episodes of antisocial, disruptive, or neglegent behavior, and a failure to function adequately with others in socially prescribed situations should be elaborated in detail since they will inevitably affect future treatment recommendations.

MENTAL STATUS EXAMINATIONS

The mental status examination is a way of organizing observational data. The purpose of the examination is to describe the patient's mental function as it appears during the interview through self descriptions. The interviewer's reactions to the patient (impressions, emotional responses, intuitive hunches) play an important part in the data collection process. Feinberg (1975) makes the point that the interviewer is both the examining instrument and the examiner, and as such should include in the assessment all personal responses to the patient. If the interviewer is confused with what originally seemed to be a straightforward account, this could be an indication of a subtlely manifested but nonetheless formal thought disorder. If the interviewer begins to feel sad at what sounds like ordinary descriptions of everyday events, this may be a first clue that the patient is depressed. Despite the subjectivity and enormity of room for error or distortion, the emotional reactions of the interviewer to the interviewee must therefore be taken into account in the assessment process.

Appearance and Behavior

Information is recorded in the mental examination according to various areas of mental functioning. During the assessment process the interviewer should note the following for recording later:

- General physical appearance. Are dress and grooming neat and appropriate? Incongruities, such as poor personal hygiene in an otherwise elegantly dressed individual, should be noted.
- Characteristic facial expressions. Does the patient maintain eye contact? Is there any facial mobility (vacant, placid, bewildered, alert, apprehensive)? Staring into space or through the interviewer as if listening or preoccupied may indicate hallucinations.
- Reactions to the interviewer. Is the patient evasive, ingratiating, overeager, cooperative, hostile, etc.?
- Motor activity. The character and amount of motor activity should be noted. Is the patient ambulatory? Is there any restlessness, mannerism, extreme slowness or motor retardation, echopraxia, or cerea flexibilitas? Are movements graceful or clumsy? Does the patient withdraw from violation of personal space?

Speech

Is the flow of language production slow and painful, as in the depressed patient, or rapid and pressured, and in manic states? Is it precise and careful, as in the obsessive or paranoid patient, or is it vague and circumlocutory, as in chronic brain syndrome? Is it coherent or is there a loosening of associations? Is there continuity or interruption of flow? Is the patient spontaneous? What level of IQ and sociocultural background does vacabulary suggest? How does the patient react to direct questions? How revealing is the patient? General speech characteristics such as tone of voice, enunciation, verbal fluency, and use of profanity should be noted. The presence of abnormalities such as incoherence, blocking, mutism, echolalia, neologisms, flight of ideas, circumstantiality, perseveration, and confabulation are important indications of mental illness.

Mood and Affect

The patient's overall feeling tone (mood) and the emotional components of the ideas expressed (affect) should be recorded. Is mood evident through body language (e.g., slumped posture in the depressed patient)? Is affect consonant with the ideas expressed? Is the range of emotional response narrowed, blunted, or flattened? Mood lability, or wide fluctuations in mood response, may be evident in patients with organic brain damage. Mood swings or any changes in the patient's affective state during the interview should be noted.

Thought Content

Thought content refers to the main themes of the interview, including the patient's concerns and preoccupations as well as content abnormalities (hallucinations, illusions, delusions, obsessions, and ideas of reference).

While delusional content is readily evident among disturbed aged patients, even more common are attributions of false, specialized, or exaggerated meanings to events that derive from personality characteristics rather than mental illness. Reported concerns may be either realistic, exaggerated, or have no discernible connection to reality.

Sensorium

Disorders of the sensorium are most often indicative of organic brain disease. Too often this aspect of the mental status examination is omitted due to either patients whose behavior appears socially appropriate (yet may mask severe brain impairment) or to the impossibility of assessing the status of the sensorium in the extremely hostile, depressed, or psychotic patient where functional disorganization of other mental processes interferes.

Orientation

Orientation to time, place, and person is routinely assessed by asking the patient if he knows who and where he is, and the date, and time. In organic brain conditions, disorientation to time precedes disorientation to place, which precedes disorientation to person. The sense of personal identity is usually the last to be lost, and recovery of orientation will occur in the reverse sequence. Of more practical concern is the ability of the aged patient to retain "pragmatic orientation" (e.g., the ability to maneuver in familiar surroundings, and to remain aware of the time to eat or sleep) since additional questions asked on most mental status quizzes such as names of presidents or state capitals will have little "survival value" for the aged isolate. Many old persons appear disoriented in unfamiliar settings such as hospitals, and a more accurate estimation of orientation would include assessing the patient's awareness of "circumstances" and ability to behave congruently with that awareness.

Memory

Thoroughly memorized material such as multiplication tables or prayers are usually retained long after the ability to abstract the meaning of proverbs is lost. To assess

- recent memory—ask what the patient had for breakfast.
- remote memory—ask about chronological events in the patient's life. These can then be compared with history data from others. Events that held great relevance for the patient will be remembered at the expense of less relevant events.
- immediate retention and recall—ask the patient to repeat three digit numbers after you—first forward, then backward, then increase to

four digit numbers. Ask the patient to repeat a name and address immediately, and again after three to five minutes.

Attention/Concentration/Arousal

Can attention be aroused and sustained? The continuum of patient response may range from hypervigilance to somnolence. Distractibility may be high. Concentration can be assessed by "serial sevens" (subtracting from 100 by sevens) or asking the patient to repeat the days of the week in reverse order.

Calculation

Ask the patient to do simple tests of calculation—serial additions, subtractions, or multiplications.

Information/Intelligence

Note the patient's vocabulary. Nonstandardized assessment measures include asking the patient to read sentences or paragraphs, then noting pronunciation and comprehension. Ask for synonyms of certain words. Ask the patient to name as many items as possible in each of the following categories—colors, fruits, animals, cities.

Insight/Judgment

Does the patient display the insight to recognize the significance of present circumstances? At the positive end of the insight continuum the neurotic knows that the source of problems is within himself, while at the negative end the psychotic fails to recognize that he is even ill.

Is the patient able to judge and compare the elements and consequences of action? Ask what the patient would do if given $10,000, or he found a stamped, addressed envelope on the street, or was lost in the woods, or smelled smoke in a movie theater.

Attitude

Describe the overall responsiveness of the patient to the assessment process. Is there neutrality, unresponsiveness, or dramatic interest? How do attitudinal shifts occur during the session? Are they in response to specific topics or circumstances?

Table 5-1 Mental Status Questionnaire

Questionnaire Items	
Question	Construct
Where are we now? Name?	Place
Where is this place located?	Place
What is today's date?	Time
What month is it?	Time
What year is it?	Time
How old are you?	Memory (recent or remote)
What is your birthday?	Memory (recent or remote)
What year were you born?	Memory (recent or remote)
Who is president of the United States?	General information memory
Who was president before him?	General information memory

Scoring	
Number of Errors	Presumed Mental Status
0–2	Chronic brain syndrome, absent or mild
3–5	Chronic brain syndrome, mild to moderate
6–8	Chronic brain syndrome, moderate to severe
9–10	Chronic brain syndrome, severe
Nontestable	Chronic brain syndrome, severe

MENTAL STATUS QUESTIONNAIRE

Cognitive impairments which derive from a final common pathways effect of varied dementing processes, produce characteristic deficits in memory, learning, and orientation. A simple and practical means of assessing the presence of such symptoms is by administration of the mental status questionnaire (MSQ) developed by Kahn, Goldfarb, Pollack, & Peck, (1960). (See Table 5-1). The test consists of ten brief questions that are easily administered and scored. The first five questions concern orientation while the second five concern general information. Scoring is simply the cumulative total of errors made. The present ten questions were reduced by means of discriminant function analysis from a larger pool of 31 questions designed to identify organic brain syndrome in elderly patients. Gurland (1980) presents an excellent, comprehensive review of the tool and its analogs (short protable MSQ), and reports test–retest reliability at 0.82 and 0.83. He also cites evidence of the tool's diagnostic validity from studies which compared it to the expert clinician's diagnostic skill. In a series of studies, when patients made no errors on the MSQ the diagnosis of chronic brain

Table 5-2 Common Psychological Tests Used in Assessment

Name of Test	Description
Babcock Examination for Efficiency of Mental Functioning	Measures vocabulary as index of mental deterioration
Bender-Gestalt Test	Measures visual-motor coordination in the detection of organic impairment
Draw-A-Person Test	Projective measurement of self-perception and body image, and as a screening device for organic impairment
Graham-Kendall Memory for Designs	Measurement of visual-motor ability and as a screening device for dementia
Halstead-Reitan Test Battery (includes W.A.I.S.)	Measurement of simple and complex motor functions, symbolic and communicative language, visual-spatial relations, abstraction and concept-formation, and general I.Q.
Halstead-Wepman Aphasia Screening Test	A battery testing or agnosias, apraxias, anomia, dysarthria and paraphasia
Index of Independence in Activities of Daily Living	Measures degree of dependence/independence in basic self-care activities
Inglis Paired Associate Learning Test	Measurement of learning/memory ability in advanced age
Life Satisfaction Index	Measures attitudes held toward quality of past, present and future life
Minesota Multiphasic Personality Inventory	Ten subscales yield a personality profile that includes, among others, measures of depression and hypochondriasis as well as psychopathological symptoms
Nurse's Observation Scale for Inpatient Evaluation	Ratings of disruptive behaviors, useful in the evaluation of the effects of treatment

Table 5-2 (*continued*)

Name of Test	Description
Philadelphia Geriatric Center Morale Scale	Measures the extent of life satisfaction versus the effects of demoralization syndrome
Wechsler Adult Intelligence Scale	Eleven subscales yield measures of verbal and performance intelligence as well as full scale I.Q. (see Chapter 6 for more detailed information)
Wechsler Memory Scale	Measurement of immediate, short-term, and long-term memory and screening for organic mental syndrome
Zung Self-Rating Depression Scale	Self-administered, brief, measurement of state as opposed to trait depression

syndrome was made independently by a geropsychiatrist in only six percent of such cases, while when patients made ten errors (the maximum possible) they were independently diagnosed as suffering from chronic organic brain syndrome in 95 percent of cases. The prognostic validity and applicability of the MSQ to health care settings is suggested by the ease of administration and the test's sensitivity to fluctuations in the patient's sensorial status. MSQ errors have been found to increase as the patient's health deteriorates. A simple loss of interest is followed by a loss of interpersonal spontaneity, declining self-care, disorientation, nonrecognition, bowel and bladder incontinence, and finally inability to eat or move, at which point maximum scores are measured. One is able therefore to estimate with some accuracy the level of nursing care needs of hospitalized patients.

ASSESSMENT TOOLS

Other commonly used assessment instruments (Table 5-2) which have revealed their differential diagnostic value in the assessment process provide invaluable data on fluctuations in the aged patient's physical and mental health status. Drawn from an increasingly broad spectrum of standardized instruments, those listed in Table 5-2 strengthen the assessment process by providing substantive data on mental deterioration, organic impairment, dementia, motor function, intelligence, dependence, depression, disruptive behavior, learning, memory, language, abstraction, concept formation, morale, and life satisfaction.

Summary

The assessment process incorporates both objective and subjective data collected by means of interview, history taking, and examination of the patient. Observation and inspection play a major role in the recording of data on verbal, nonverbal, and behavioral aspects of mental status. Mental process in advanced age often reflects the interactive effects of bodily, personal or social dysfunction. Symptoms of both psychogenic and physiogenic etiology can be viewed as manifestations of a final common pathway.

The development of a psychodiagnostic formulation necessitates consideration of specific questions to be included in the assessment plan and in evaluation of assessment findings. The interviewer's orientation to the process and the patient will have appreciable effect on what and how material is noted. History taking should include a thorough medical, historical, personal, familial, and social compilation of facts and impressions that will facilitate the identification of specific goals for intervention, and their means of attainment.

The mental status examination will cover the patient's general appearance and behavior, speech and communication practices, general mood and emotional expressions, thought processes and content, and specific indicators of intact versus dysfunctional sensorium. The mental status questionnaire, particularly applicable to assessment of geriatric mental process, is but one of many psychometric instruments that can be used in the comprehensive assessment of the aged.

REFERENCES

Feinberg, I. (1975). The psychiatric work-up. In I. Glick (Ed.), *Syllabus–Introduction to clinical psychiatry* (pp. 5–18). San Francisco: University of California.

Freedman, A., Kaplan, H., & Sadock, B. (1976). *Modern synopsis of comprehensive textbook of psychiatry/II*. Baltimore: Williams and Wilkins Co.

Gurland, B. (1980). The assessment of the mental health status of older adults. In J. Birren & R. Sloane (Eds.), *Handbook of mental health and aging* (pp. 671–700). Englewood Cliffs, NJ: Prentice-Hall.

Kahn, R., Goldfarb, A., Pollack, M., & Peck, A. (1960). Brief objective measures for the determination of mental status in the aged. *American Journal of Psychiatry, 117*, 326–328.

Lomax, J. (1982). Psychotherapy of psychophysiological disorders. In W. Fann, I. Karacan, A. Pokorny, & R. Williams (Eds.), *Phenomenology and treatment of psychophysiological disorders* (pp. 251–258). New York: Spectrum Publications, Inc.

Small, L. (1973). *Neuropsychodiagnosis in psychotherapy*. New York: Brunner/Mazel.

SUGGESTED READINGS

Eaton, M., & Petersen, M. (1969). *Psychiatry*. New York: Medical Examination Publishing Company.

Solomon, P. & Sturrock, J. (1974). The psychiatric examination. In P. Solomon & V. Patch (Eds.), *Handbook of psychiatry* (pp. 26–49). Los Altos, CA: Lange Medical Publications.

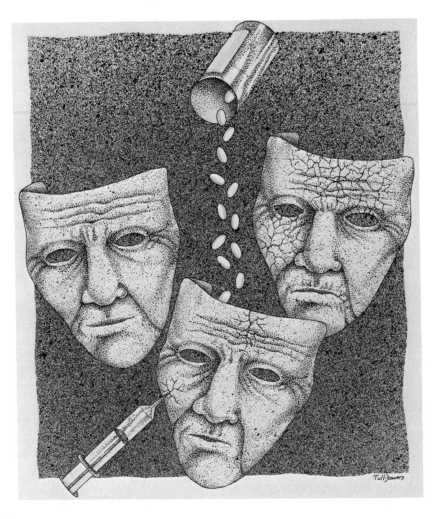

Chapter 6

Assessing the Interaction of Mind and Body

The interaction of mind and body is complex and still poorly understood. Increased mortality rates from loneliness or bereavement, although well documented, fail to explain the exact mechanisms by which intellect and emotion may activate terminal physiological mechanisms and bring about death. We know that it can happen, but are at a loss to explain just how.

Interaction between various systems of the body is so extensive that any change in one system inevitably brings about a change in others. Changes in the endocrine system activate changes in sensory awareness and acuity. Changes in the central nervous system result in altered psychomotor function, behavior, personality, and emotions. Changes in intellectual and cognitive functioning are commonly attributed to decreased cerebrovascular activity, which may also cause changes in motivation and language. We know that intellect is dependent upon adequate cerebral blood flow but what role do fluctuating levels of choline, acetylcholine, and monoamine oxidase play?

This chapter attempts to address one part of this dilemma by examining various systemic changes that present as neuropsychiatric symptomatology, even though each change is of pathophysiological etiology. At present there are almost 1,000 known causes of reversible senile dementia-like symptoms, the result of potentially treatable disease. Changes in mentation result from cardiovascular, renal, hematopoietic, gastrointestinal, metabolic, endocrine, or nutritional disorders, to name but a few. For example, at age 80 the interaction of stress and pulmonary function is evident in a 50 percent reduction in oxygen consumption.

The author wishes to acknowledge the assistance of Susan Smith R.N., M. S. and Brenda Jackson R.N., M.S., whose help was invaluable in the preparation of this chapter.

A multiplicity of interactions occur: aging and disease; aging, disease, and CNS activity; overt disease and covert, preexisting disorder; and the interaction of aging, disease, drugs, nutrition and stress. Physical and mental reserves are lowered in the elderly, and this predisposes them to a greater variety of nonspecific manifestations of illness than in younger age groups, and increases their vulnerability to progressive, deteriorative psychiatric disorders. Systemic diseases in this age group frequently lead to nonspecific, imprecise and fluctuating mental symptoms. When left undiagnosed and untreated, relatively simple medical problems deteriorate into secondary and tertiary complications in much the same way that acute reversible brain syndrome will deteriorate into irreversible chronic brain syndrome if untreated.

Early detection, and a diagnosis made with awareness of multiple causation, is crucial to the prevention of mental deterioration. The elderly have tended to underreport illness, suggesting that when they finally enter the health care system secondary and tertiary effects may be in evidence. The reverse may also be true; that the presenting symptoms have little to do with underlying pathological processes. Contemporary estimates suggest that between 10 and 30 percent of the geriatric population develop mental symptoms as a result of unrecognized, potentially treatable diseases (Anderson, 1966). The necessity for thorough and precise assessment of mental and physical status is clear.

NEUROPSYCHIATRIC MANIFESTATIONS OF PHYSICAL DISORDERS

Manifestations of Cardiovascular Disease

Greater attention is being paid to the interaction of cardiac disease and psychiatric symptomatology. The relationship between the two is no longer considered to be unidirectional, since disturbances of heart function, and vascular disease, may result in a variety of cerebral changes with behavioral manifestations. The following are fairly common symptoms of mental disorder of cardiovascular etiology.

Intermittent Confusion. Cardiac malfunction may result in a generalized reduction in cerebral blood flow of acute or chronic nature. Changes both in cardiac conduction and intrinsic heart rate may lead to signs of mental fatigue and intermittent confusion. Confusion may also result from vascular disease. Increased peripheral resistance may lead to increased perfusion pressure required for tissues. Impaired oxygenation, vascular inability to provide nutrients (glucose) and remove metabolic wastes, and decreased cerebral blood flow, may all induce episodic confusion.

Acute Confusion. Acute confusional states may result from cerebral embolization from the heart, with selective destruction or infarction of parts of the brain. Showers of micro-emboli from calcifications on aortic and mitral valves, as well as small blood clots on rigid valve surfaces, may lead to cerebral dysfunction and confusion.

Disorientation. Chronic hypoxia resulting from congestive heart failure may reduce levels of consciousness and orientation.

Intellectual Deficiency. Tissues of the brain are extremely sensitive to oxygen deficit and may be seriously damaged following cardiac arrest. Because of inequality in brain sensitivity to hypoxia (the cerebral cortex is considerably less resistent than vegetative structures of the brainstem), recovery from cardiac arrest may reveal normal vegetative functions but permanent intellectual deficiency.

Loss of Consciousness. Dizziness, blackouts, or syncope may result from cardiac conduction defects such as heart block or arrhythmia which decrease cardiac output. Syncope may also result from reflex asystole or atherosclerosis of vertibral arteries and/or the carotid artery.

Memory Loss. Loss of memory may occur as a result of hypertension or other deteriorative vascular disease in which deficits in oxygen and tissue regeneration are crucial.

Depression. Depressive symptoms may be considered likely following cardiac insult, and are increasingly being considered a significant precipitating factor as well.

Drug Effects. Antihypertensive agents may reduce needed cerebral perfusion pressure and reduce cerebral blood flow, causing confusion. Cardioactive agents such as digitalis may induce toxicity that results in confusion, disorientation, irritability, stupor, hallucinations, and psychosis, in addition to visual disturbances such as amblyopia, diplopia, or blurring, each of which is also disorientating.

Nonspecific Organic Brain Syndrome. According to Rosenberg (1981), cardiovascular conditions that induce a generalized reduction in cerebral blood flow, and over all impairment of brain function, are not easily differentiated from each other or from other toxic or metabolic processes on the basis of observed effects. Consequently, all may produce nonspecific organic brain syndrome.

Manifestations of Renal Disease

The common tendency of older adults to underreport illness, one initially described by Anderson (1966) as a result of research on illness reporting behavior in Scotland, provided us with valuable data. Underreporting illness allows delayed, altered, and secondary manifestations to combine with age-related changes in renal function, and when this occurs it may predispose the elderly patient to fluid and electrolyte imbalance. Disorders of electrolyte imbalance, particularly saltwater balance and potassium level, when combined with the diminished mental reserves of the aged, can result in the presentation of neuropsychiatric symptoms.

Hypernatremia. Hypernatremia is a hyperosmolarity syndrome secondary to inadequate fluid intake, disphoresis without fluid replacement, cerebral injury, or iatrogenic factors such as IV or intraperitoneal administration of hypertonic saline or tube-feeding high-protein mixtures. A common reluctance of dehydrated elderly patients to drink often compounds the problem, since their impaired level of consciousness may block an already blunted thirst mechanism. Regardless of cause, the clinical effects of hypernatremia manifest themselves as depression of the central nervous system with resultant lethargy and acute confusional episodes. Common neuromuscular abnormalities include muscle rigidity, tremor, and seizures. Diffuse EEG abnormalities may be present, and confusion may deepen progressively into coma.

Hyponatremia. Hyponatremia is a hypo-osmolarity syndrome secondary to increased antidiuretic hormone (ADA) secretion or other possible conditions such as pneumonia or congestive heart failure. A disorder of water intoxication, it is perhaps the most serious and least well recognized electrolyte disorder in the elderly. Imbalance between gain in brain water versus loss of brain electrolytes (intracerebral potassium and/or sodium) may result in symptoms such as those reported by Minaker and Rowe (1981). They found symptoms of aberrant taste or thirst, insomnia, nightmares, lethargy, muscle fatigue and cramping, deja vu experiences, stupor, acute psychosis, and in more acute cases coma and death. For one group studied, mortality was reported at 50 percent, in spite of individualized treatment supervision. Several of these studies have demonstrated a significant correlation between level of hyponatremia and degree of depressed sensorium.

Hypokalemia. Hypokalemia is caused by a disturbance of potassium balance that may be etiologically attributed to inadequate potassium intake, diaphoresis, dilution of extracellular fluid volume, shift in intracellular potassium, excess gastrointestinal loss via vomiting or diarrhea, pituitary–adrenal disturbance, renal disorder, idiopathic cause. In addition, the elderly are frequent recipients of drugs that have been shown to induce this syndrome. Neuromuscular weakness is characteristic, and with decreases in total body potassium, common psychiatric symptoms such as altered levels of consciousness, lethargy, apathy, drowsiness, irritability, confusion and occasionally coma, delirium, and hallucinations may all be present.

Hyperkalemia. Hyperkalemia appears only in association with acute renal failure, excessive potassium supplementation resulting from thiazide diuretic therapy, severe acidosis, or deficiencies of aldosterone or cortisol. Clinical symptoms which are subtle and appear late in the course of illness include anxiety, restlessness, apprehension, weakness, and stupor. Monitoring of potassium supplementation in elderly patients on thiazide diuretics is crucial to the prevention of potentially lethal hyperkalemia, since symptoms may appear only shortly before cardiac arrhythmias, which may cause death.

Uremia. Literature on psychiatric manifestations of uremia is scant, but Minaker and Rowe (1981) report that 75 percent of a large series of acute and chronic uremic patients experienced psychiatric symptoms when BUN levels exceeded 250 mg/dl, while another 60 percent with BUN levels between 50–199 mg/dl exhibited mental dysfunction. With progressive renal failure, characteristic symptoms include fatigue, fluctuations in mental state, drowsiness, inability to concentrate, apathy, altered appetite, decreased libido, depression, and irritability. Sleep patterns may be reversed. Paranoid behaviors are fairly common. Paradoxical euphoria may develop and delirious psychosis may increase, while general mental ability declines.

Drug Therapy. Drug therapy, particularly diuretic therapies, must be closely monitored since the reduced ability of the kidney to clear drugs may easily lead to a prolonged half-life of certain agents, may precipitate serious fluid and electrolyte imbalance, and may produce symptoms of mental deterioration through the mechanisms of dehydration, hyperosmolarity, uremia, hyperglycemia, hyponatremia, or hypopotassemia.

Lower Urinary Tract Disease. Involuntary loss of urine, difficult voiding, frequency of voiding, and nocturia may all induce psychological and psychiatric symptoms such as intense anxiety (from a fear of involuntary voiding), compulsive self-protection (from discovery by others of wet spots on clothing or inordinate periods of time spent in the bathroom), frustration (from the extent to which frequency of urination interferes with work routine and productivity), irritability (from sleep that is continually interrupted due to frequent nocturia), depression (from the cumulative effects of anxiety, embarrassment, and frustration), and delusions (that the individual constantly smells of urine or is continually wet).

Manifestations of Hematopoietic Disease

Hematologic system disease may present psychiatric symptoms through profound effect on the central nervous system. According to Weinger (1981) these effects take place when oxygen transport and delivery is decreased, abnormal hemostasis causes intracerebral hemorrhage, blood cell production or nerve tissue metabolism is deficient, malignant cell proliferation involves certain nerves, products of cell proliferation alter blood properties, or immunological defects predispose to central nervous system infections.

Vitamin B₁₂ Deficiency. The role of Vitamin B_{12} in psychiatric illness in old age remains unclear, but psychiatric manifestations have been described (Weinger, 1981). The clinical symptoms may include personality change, depression, dementia, memory or intellectual impairment, abnormal EEG findings, and confusion. These symptoms may also be present in the absence of anemia.

CNS Leukemia. A specific psychiatric syndrome accompanying CNS leukemia has not been described, but "metabolic" psychosis has been found to occur, with altered states of consciousness, confusion, and/or personality change in evidence.

Hyperviscosity. A hyperviscosity syndrome, the result of accumulations in the serum of excessive amounts of immunoglobulin protein, has been described (Weinger, 1981) as presenting a variable and confusing picture. Symptoms such as weakness, easy fatigability, anorexia, headache, transient paresis, paresthesias, vertigo, confusion, and coma may occur.

Progressive Multifocal Leukoencephalopathy (PML). PML occurs in patients with associated immune deficits, usually in those with underlying leukemia or lymphoma, and is apparently the result of a DNA infection. Symptoms include impaired awareness and disorientation, lessened general mental abilities, and abnormal emotional responses.

Manifestations of Respiratory Disease

Because of the vital gas exchange role of the lungs, certain respiratory and extrapulmonary abnormalities may present as states of confusion or other psychiatric symptoms. Chronic infection may induce an insidious general mental and physical decline, while carcinoma may induce mental deterioration through metastasis. In addition, the following conditions may induce mental change.

Hyperventilation. Hyperventilation, a disease usually associated with youth, can in the acute form result in respiratory alkalosis, with a profound decrease in cerebral blood flow. A 40 percent decrement in blood flow has been demonstrated following only several minutes of overbreathing. According to Hall (1981) such a decrement is hardly surprising in the elderly, whose cerebral blood flow may be already sufficiently compromised to induce varied central nervous system manifestations. Symptoms of hyperventilation include irritability, agitation, sleep disturbance, nightmares, apprehension, inability to concentrate, light headedness, and dizziness.

Pulmonary Embolic Disease. Pulmonary embolic disease can result from diminished physical activity and prolonged periods of bedrest. Findings from several investigations (Hall, 1981) have indicated that most of the 50,000 deaths annually in the United States from pulmonary embolism are among persons over age 70. Nonspecific and frequently overlooked mental symptoms include acute anxiety attacks, apprehension, agitation, and even panic.

Pneumonia, Hypoxia, and Hypercapnia. Pneumonia, hypoxia and hypercapnia may influence preexisting, age-dependent declines in arterial PO_2, already compromised oxygen delivery, and may increase susceptibility of the brain to lowered oxygen availability. Resulting symptoms include altered behavior patterns, paranoia, disturbances of consciousness, confusion, agitation, and markedly impaired judgement. These may occur in the absence of focal neurological manifestations.

Chronic Obstructive Pulmonary Disease (COPD). COPD in the aged is often characterized by depreciation of the ailment by the patient. Chronic cough and sputum production may be overlooked. The patient has been frequently isolated at home and possibly depressed, but these factors may not be initially associated with COPD. Clinical symptoms include denial, depression, rage reaction, mild sedation, combativeness, agitation, and disorientation, all of which may coexist within the individual.

Manifestations of Gastrointestinal Disease

Liver disease and its consequent effect upon mental function has been quite widely reported in the literature (Hoffman, 1981). Cirrhosis, obstruction of the bile ducts with subsequent elevation of plasma bilirubin, and inflamation of the liver have all been shown to include the possibility of some mental status change. Vitamin deficiency and metabolic disorder also influence gastrointestinal changes that may in turn result in mental symptoms.

Chronic Hepatitis. Although the incidence is very slight, chronic hepatitis may present with confusional symptoms.

Intestinal Obstruction. Mental confusion may result from intestinal obstruction of varied cause, including fecal impaction (which is common among immobilized, chronically ill patients).

Gastrointestinal Bleeding. Deterioration of mental status from upper or lower tract bleeding as well as from aspirin-induced hemorrhagic gastritis, gastric ulcer, or esophageal varices, has been reported among elderly patients (Lavis, 1981).

Carcinoma of the Pancreas. Depression has been found to be a major symptom and sometimes the most common mental change associated with the course of the disease in the aged.

Vitamin Deficiency. Vitamin B_{12} deficiency has already been mentioned as etiologically associated with mental changes in old age, and some researchers believe that deficiencies of vitamin B_{12} may be a principal cause of dementia (Altman, Mehta, Evenson, & Sletten, 1973). Deficiencies of other vitamins, such as A and C, as well as thiamine and riboflavin, have been accompanied by alterations in mental function. Symptoms such as depression, apathy, irritability, confusion, and delirium have all been reported (Gershell, 1981). Thiamine deficiency, seen in Korsakoff's syndrome, may cause memory deficit and confabulation. Niacin deficiency, extremely rare in our society, is known to induce the characteristic four D's; dermatitis, diarrhea, dementia, and death (with symptoms arising in that order).

Chronic Liver Disease with Porto-Systemic Encephalopathy (PSE). The primary cause of PSE is alcoholic liver disease, with a fairly high incidence among men in their fifth and sixth decades. Cryptogenic cirrhosis is also likely among the elderly, and it may present as PSE. The PSE syndrome is attributed to a portal-to-systemic venous shunt, with the collection of nitrogenous material in the gastrointestinal tract. According to Hoffman (1981), a clinical picture emerges that is manifested by altered mental status, neuromuscular symptoms, and fetor hepaticus (sweet or musty breath odor). Mood alterations, euphoria, or depression may all occur, but euphoria is more common. Disturbed sleep pattern, stupor, and coma may follow. Several theories have attempted to explain the etiology and course of the disease, but it is now commonly accepted that each cause ultimately results, either directly or indirectly, in interference with normal neurotransmission in the central nervous system.

Acute Intermittent Porphyria. Acute intermittent porphyria is a rare metabolic disorder characterized by physical (abdominal pain, constipation) and neuropsychiatric symptoms. Etiological mechanisms inducing the disorder are complex and not fully understood, but mental symptoms include depression, confusion, hallucinations and disorientation.

Manifestations of Endocrine Disease

Because of the degree of systemic interaction associated with aging, the classic symptoms of endocrine disease may be modified or even absent in the elderly. Somatic signs and symptoms may be unreliable, or they may resemble degenerative manifestations such as those found in organic brain syndrome. Due to the elusive character of symptoms of endocrine disorder in the elderly, reliance upon laboratory testing is strongly recommended. A metabolic screening battery has been recommended by Lavis (1981) as essential to adequate endocrine diagnosis, and should include fasting serum glucose, serum calcium, serum sodium, serum thyroxine, resin T3 uptake, and in men, serum testosterone. While descriptive data on psychiatric symptoms of specific endocrinopathies are limited, understanding of the relationship between them has increased. The interdependence of mentation capacity, the endocrine system, and the central nervous system is suggested by certain clinical phenomena.

Hypothalamus–Pituitary Complex. Hypofunction of the pituitary gland may result in mental confusion, while a decrease in hypothalamic stimulating hormones (catecholamines and other neurotransmitters, such as norepinephrine, which is both hormone and neurotransmitter) may be related to depressive states.

Hyperthyroidism. Contrary to the common clinical stereotype of hyperthyroidism among younger persons, hyperthyroidism among the elderly may present symptoms such as apathy, anorexia, constipation, depression, or dementia. Hyperkinetic excitement, restlessness, and irritability are uncommon in the aged patient with hyperthyroid disorder.

Hypothyroidism. Hypothyroidism offers the classical syndrome by which many elderly patients are diagnosed as having dementia. Characteristic symptoms include weakness, apathy, depression, slower mental and physical responsiveness, loss of auditory acuity, lethargy, intolerance to cold, drying of the skin, paresthesias, paranoia, and delirium. In some instances thyroxine replacement therapy will affect mental and physical improvements, while in other instances mental status will remain unchanged.

Hyperparathyroidism. Primary hyperparathyroidism results in the overproduction and overactivity of parathyroid hormone, and is present in hypercalcemia, a condition also associated with neuropsychiatric symptomatology. Various organs are involved in hyperparathyroidism, including bones, kidneys, gastrointestinal tract and the central nervous system. Karpati and Frame (1964) have reported neuropsychiatric disorders related to hyperparathyroidism that include confusion, disorientation, fluctuating levels of consciousness, and frequent sensorial clouding.

Hypoparathyroidism. Hypoparathyroidism is an abnormally decreased production of parathyroid hormone that causes hypocalcemia. Decreased parathyroid hormone, the result of thyroidectomy or idiopathic etiology, has also been associated with characteristic reversible mental changes such as confusion, disorientation, and clouded sensorium, seen in pseudosenility.

Hypercalcemia. Hypercalcemia has multiple etiologies, but frequently appears secondary to hyperparathyroidism. It may also be secondary to carcinoma of the lung, breast, or other tissue, multiple myeloma, Paget's disease coupled with immobilization, thiazide administration, vitamin D intoxication, milk–alkali syndrome, Addison's disease or thyroid dysfunction. Clinical symptoms include fatigue, muscle weakness, constipation, anorexia, and at times cardiac arrhythmia. The incidence of hypercalcemia among the elderly is fairly high and neuropsychiatric symptoms develop insidiously, frequently being attributed to other pathological processes. A strong positive correlation between abnormal plasma level of calcium and mental deterioration has not been established, since plasma levels of 12–13 mg/dl may produce confusion in a patient, while in another 14–15 mg/dl may not. Recent research has been accumulating that documents the presence of increased cerebral calcium in states of sustained hyperparathyroidism, suggesting direct or indirect sensitivity of the brain to parathyroid hormone (Cogan, Covey, Arieff, et al., 1978; Karpati & Frame, 1964). Additional evidence supports the premise of "paracrine" systems within the brain in which, according to Lavis (1981), specific neurotransmitter–hormonal peptides such as somatostatin are synthesized and released by neurons to act on neighboring cells.

Variation in mental symptomatology may relate to rapidity of fluctuation in serum levels. The neuropsychiatric manifestations of fluctuating calcium levels may be described as severe alterations in mental functions. These include fluctuations in level of confusion, orientation, consciousness, retardation, or fatigue, plus involuntary tremors or choreiform movements.

Hypocalcemia. Hypocalcemia usually occurs secondary to hypoparathyroidism, malabsorptive states, or renal failure. A reduction in ionization of calcium results in increased irritability, and spontaneous discharge of sensory and motor nerves and muscle, producing paresthesias, twitching, and muscular spasms (tetany). Most patients are not weak, but those with primary hypoparathyroidism may develop muscle weakeness proximal to the midline. Improvement usually follows treatment with calcium and vitamin D. Hypocalcemia may also result from osmotic diarrhea, induced by administration of potassium-depleting diuretics. Neuropsychiatric symptoms of pseudosenility, mentioned previously, compound existing neuromuscular and sensorimotor findings.

Hypoglycemia. Hypoglycemia may have an onset that is mild and clinically undiagnosed, producing progressive mental deterioration. If the hypoglycemic state is severe, extented, or repeated, it may lead to irreversible brain damage. Confusion, lethargy, and dementia are symptomatic. Hypoglycemia may also occur rapidly and without symptoms of increased sympathetic nervous system activity (diaphoresis, tachycardia, tachypnea). Coma may occur without warning. Episodic bizarre behavior, slurring of speech, disorientation, confusion, somnolence, and difficult arousal must be considered symptomatic in the elderly diabetic receiving insulin or oral hypoglycemic agents.

Hyperglycemia. Characteristic symptoms of the ketoacidotic state are well known, making it relatively easy to diagnose. Less easily detected, and almost unique to the elderly, is a severe hypoglycemic syndrome in the absence of ketosis–nonketotic hyperosmolarity syndrome, which progresses gradually either undiagnosed or occurs in previously well controlled patients. Characteristic neuropsychiatric symptoms include confusion, stupor, and coma.

Manifestations of Central Nervous System Disorders

The central nervous system is a dynamic system capable of significant adaptation. It has a vast reserve capacity which allows selection of response to stimuli, behavioral variation, and even loss of substance without severely altering function. Many of the disorders of old age are attributable to neurological deficits. Drachman (1980) has reported findings indicating that neurological disorders are the most common cause of disability in the elderly, accounting for almost half of the incapacities after age 65, and for over 90 percent of serious dependencies.

As has been previously demonstrated, the central nervous system plays a pivotal role in the health of all body systems. This is particularly so in effecting subtle, interactive changes that present as mental or behavioral rather than physical disorders. Much of this symptomatic subtlety can be traced to age-related physiological alterations, including a loss of brain substance, decrease of gyri, loss of nerve cells, widening of sulci, reduction of white matter, and loss of brain weight. The system is composed exclusively of postmitotic neuronal elements, so that some degree of deterioration is inevitable over time. Age-related systemic changes and diseases combine to produce alterations in neurological, psychological and emotional functions.

Altered Neurological Function

Altered neurological function may result from each of the following conditions, all presenting with overt manifestations of pseudosenility.

Tumors. According to Libow (1973) intracranial tumors present with behavioral alterations in 50-70 percent of cases. Symptoms may be delayed due to increased available intracranial space, the result of cerebral atrophy. Almost half of all tumors seen in this age group are metastases from carcinoma of the lung or breast.

Aphasia. Pseudosenile behaviors may be associated with the inability to transmit or receive ideas through any form of language, due to partial or complete loss of ability to deal with the known symbols of language.

Normal Pressure Hydrocephalus. The underlying cause of this compensated hydrocephalus is thought to be a failure of absorption of cerebrospinal fluid (CSF) due to fibrotic changes in the meninges and arachnoid granulations following either subarachnoid hemorrhage, trauma, or meningeal inflammation. Normal or nearly normal pressure is maintained, possibly due to the ventricles within the skull enlarging at the expense of cerebral tissue, until pressure is stabilized at an equilibrium between the rate of production and the rate of absorption of CSF. Characteristic symptoms of dementia may be relieved by surgical shunting of CSF from the ventricles to the peritoneal cavity.

Parkinsonism. Although etiologically ideopathic, estimates of mental impairment with Parkinsonism range from 25–80 percent. Characteristic mental symptoms include a sensorial dulling or apathetic obtundity, and an overt inability to initiate response. General mental deterioration has been halted by treatment with l-Dopa, but mental and physical improvement with l-Dopa is temporary and the drug has itself been associated with dementia-like adverse effects.

Infections. Confusional states, disorientation, and clouded sensorium have all been associated with meningitis, brain abscess, and herpes simplex encephalities.

Altered Psychological Function

Altered psychological functions that reflect underlying cerebral substance disorders frequently present with manifestations characteristic of organic dementia, which may masquerade as a functional psychosis, an emotional liability, or an accentuation or exaggeration of previous personality characteristics. Behavioral changes associated with each of the following conditions may, however, present as manifestations of either functional or organic mental disorder.

Rigidity of Response. A loss of adaptability and increase in fixed response patterns by the aged results in stereotyped behavior. The need for rigidity of reaction to stimuli reflects their need for stability of environmental conditions. New settings and new circumstances may precipitate confusion that is behaviorally evident in a confused stream of thought, easy distractability, and inability to disregard extraneous details.

Misinterpretation of Environmental Stimuli. Misinterpretation of environmental stimuli is a concomitant of organic dementia, but it is also a reflection of altered sensory acuity, age-related change in reactivity, and intolerance of neural noise. The normal ability to differentiate and discard the multiplicity of insignificant stimuli which impinge on us from the environment is reduced with age. Fragmented conversation or distal noise may easily be misinterpreted as "voices" and lead to suspiciousness or paranoia. The problem is further compounded by decreased visual, auditory, or tactile acuity, and insufficient feedback from within the environment itself to enable reorientation.

Depression. Depression is common in the elderly. Reduced psychomotor and mental activity often make it difficult to distinguish depression from organic mental syndrome. Multiple economic, social, and psychological losses frequently lead to regressed behavior and preoccupation with an internal world.

Immobilization. Immobilization, particularly in institutional settings, reduces the degree of sensory stimulation available to the aged patient and can induce metabolic changes that affect all organ functions. Any organic damage that is present may be worsened by sensory deprivation, which can lead to regressive behavior that is characterized by apathy, withdrawal, fear, panic reactions, and inchoate or complete loss of speech.

Altered Emotional Function

Altered emotional reactions associated with central nervous system disorders are frequently characterized by labile instability. The cortical theory of emotional etiology holds that emotions arise from the hippocampi, are transferred to the mamillary bodies, continue to the anterior thalamic nuclei, from which they radiate to the cortex of the cingulate gyri. The theory provides an explanation of how emotions arise as a result of excitation of either the cortical or hypothalamic levels. Emotions are associated with frontal lobe function as well as limbic system circuitry. The prefrontal regions of the brain are concerned with foresight, imagination, and self-appreciation. According to Fields (1981), each of these psychological functions is invested with emotion via association pathways that link the hypothalamus and cingulate gyri of the cerebral hemispheres to the thalami and hippocampi. Functions of this part of the brain are directed to adjustment of the whole personality to future contingencies. The ability to be alert and prepared for the unexpected, which may intrude abruptly, is located here. Though the precise mechanisms are still not fully understood, direct or indirect insult to this region of the brain results in the type of emotional instability that is so commonly seen in neurologically impaired individuals. Diffuse lesions are even more likely to evoke extreme emotional responses to almost any emotional stimuli.

Cerebrovascular Disease. Precipitate anger, irritability, fear, depression, crying, apprehension, and volatile mood swings totally out of proportion to the occasion are commonly observed in patients with cerebrovascular disease.

Organic Brain Disease. Combativeness, aggressiveness, deep depressive withdrawal, apathy, euphoria, hyperanxiety, and abrupt alterations in mood are frequently observed in patients with organic brain disease. Emotional lability may be so marked that emotional patterns change from day to day or even from hour to hour. Depression, however, seems to be more common among individuals of a cyclothymic temperament whose premorbid personality held preexisting tendencies to it.

Illness. The impact of illness alone precipitates fear and uncertainty. For the socially traumatized elderly, anger and bewilderment may be normal reactions. Facing the unknown evokes a natural anxiety, and the threat of unknown danger ahead *should* instill a protective degree of apprehension. Yet, suspecting that one suffers from some degree of brain damage can evoke even greater emotional turmoil that seriously undermines the emotional equilibrium of the aged patient.

Manifestations of Nutritional Deficiency

The association between mental deterioration and vitamin deficiency has been studied closely in recent years with ever more provocative findings. A recent United States Senate Subcommittee on Aging (1976) investigation revealed that a third to a half of all health problems of the aged could be traced to the direct consequences of nutritional disorder, malnutrition, or obesity. Even marginal or preclinical vitamin deficiencies can lead to nonspecific symptoms such as malaise, irritability, sonmolence, loss of appetite and weight, and impaired psychological and physical performance. The manner in which nutrition status affects true dementia remains unclear, but researchers like Gershell (1981) believe that subclinical deficiencies probably help to precipitate confusional states in the frail elderly whose homeostatic balance is already impaired. The high incidence of intermittent confusional states among the elderly raises the possibility that inadequate nutrition may be a widespread causative factor of mental deterioration. Significant findings linking specific deficiencies to aberrant mental symptoms are appearing with increasing frequency in the literature (Altman, et al., 1973).

Marginal Vitamin Deficiencies. Marginal deficiencies, if undiagnosed and untreated, have been found to result in severe weight loss, cachexia, iron deficiency, anemias, folate deficiency, scurvy, and osteomalacia, all of which may present as episodic confusion and disorientation.

Iron Deficiency. Iron deficiency anemia is widespread among the elderly and is due mainly to inadequate diet or malabsorption. Behavioral symptoms include weakness, apathy, and lack of appetite and initiative.

Vitamin B$_{12}$ Deficiency. This deficiency has been discussed previously as a factor in hematopoietic and gastrointestinal disorders that yield psychiatric symptomatology, but sufficient data exist (Gershell, 1981) to support the conclusion that a deficiency can cause organic brain syndrome and other functional psychiatric disorders. If left untreated, irreversible brain damage is possible. A broad spectrum of psychiatric symptoms has been reported in the absence of subacute combined degeneration, or the abnormality of peripheral blood or bone marrow. Anemia need not be present in concert with B_{12} abnormality, or positive mental or neurological findings. Another study found a high correlation between low serum B_{12} and a high incidence of psychiatric disorders (Gershell, 1981). The deficiency should be suspected in any obscure mental or neurological disorder in the aged regardless of anemia, since therapeutic dosages of B_{12} may correct the anemia but fail to resolve the neuropsychiatric symptoms due to irreversible demyelinization of areas of the cerebral cortex.

Folate Deficiency. Research on true folate deficiency has yielded findings that are highly variable (Gershell, 1981). Folate deficiency has been found among 60–80 percent of subject samples and controls in geropsychiatric and nursing home settings. Mental symptoms tend to be mild and nonspecific, with apathy and depression commonly observed.

Pyridoxine (Vitamin B_6) Deficiency. Although the incidence of pyridoxine deficiency among the elderly is quite low, in cases of fairly mild deficiency symptoms of anorexia, depression, confusion, lassitude, and weakness have preceded somatic complaints.

Zinc Deficiency. Deficiencies of zinc have been reported to lead to diminished sensations of taste and smell, sensory diminutions that could easily impair appetite in the elderly. Deficiencies of zinc are believed by some investigators to be as common and as important as the widespread deficiencies of iron and vitamin C.

Alcohol and Diet. Alcoholism among the aged has been recognized as a serious problem, the manifestations of which are often confused with malnutrition, with symptoms similar to Korsakoff's and Wernicke's syndromes. Since the older chronic alcoholic is frequently diagnosed as a mental patient with organic brain syndrome and admitted to a psychiatric hospital, diagnostic vigilance is crucial. Organic brain syndrome is often reversible if detected and treated promptly. Alcohol toxicity in the aged may present an acute onset with altered levels of awareness, mild confusion, and a progressive stupor that leads to acute delirium. The patient's disorientation and impaired intellectual functions may mimic chronic, irreversible brain syndrome. Unless properly diagnosed, these untreated, reversible brain syndromes can merge into a chronic and irreversible state.

Both alcoholics with presenting psychiatric symptoms and elderly patients with mental deterioration frequently exhibit lower-than-normal blood levels of vitamin C. A ''neurotic triad'' has been reported by Kinsman and Hood (1971) that is characterized by hypochondriases, depression, and hysteria as accompaniment to moderate ascorbic acid deficiency. Among psychogeriatric inpatients, Altman and associates, (1973) reported that six weeks of multivitamin supplementation produced a statistically significant reduction in pathological manifestations of alcoholism. Psychometric assessment revealed a dramatic decline for nonschizophrenic patients in comparison to the control groups. The findings from both studies reinforce the need for careful assessment of the nutritional and mental status of the aged patient.

Depression. The frequency of depression as a neuropsychiatric symptom has been discussed previously, but it is worth noting that depression is often involved in a vicious cycle with nutritional disorders in old age. It is unlikely that any single nutritional deficiency exists at any one point in time. Instead, because several systems undergo decline or pathological change simultaneously, it is far more likely that multiple deficiencies coexist, creating a generalized loss of energy. Depression and malnutrition then exacerbate each other; limited energy and mobility leads to a loss of initiative, which in turn leads to a loss of appetite and depression, which subsequently reduces sustenance intake. The syndrome is similar to marasmus and "failure to thrive" syndrome seen in infants deprived of affective ties. This must be taken into consideration when assessing the elderly, particularly those living alone.

Manifestations of Drugs, Trauma, Surgery and Stress

Drugs

Drugs are now widely known to cause insidious and severe changes in the physical and mental well-being of the elderly. Chapter 10 addresses in depth the role played by chemotherapeutic agents. What warrants mentioning here are several points that bear upon the vulnerability of the aged to drug-induced neuropsychiatric manifestations. As the leading consumers of drugs in our society, the number of errors in self-medicating practice by the elderly has increased alarmingly in recent years. Labels with fine print too small to be read, pills that resemble each other, visual acuity that fluctuates, and a mind that forgets, leave the aged open to mistakes that can have profound consequences.

The cost of prescription drugs, and the well-advertized availability of over-the-counter substitutes, make self-medicating a sensible, if potentially lethal, temptation. Polypharmacy, abuse of nonprescription drugs, and age-related physiological changes that potentiate drug sensitivity, create causative aggregates that result in rather tragic effects.

The ease with which confusion and disorientation can occur in the absence of prescription and nonprescription drugs only serves to heighten the acute sensitivity of the aged to all foreign substances. Their own physiological predisposition to ideopathic pseudodementia places them in the unique position of being so vulnerable that injudicious drug use does little more than virtually guarantee secondary psychiatric complications.

Trauma

Confusion, disorientation, and mental deterioration are commonly seen in elderly patients following trauma. Aberrant behavior, such as inappropriate aggression and combativeness, or extreme apathy, is often seen following head trauma or subarachnoid hemorrhage. Accidental falls are common in the aged, and the resultant subdural hematomas may be diagnosed only by the clinical presentation of fluctuating consciousness, confusion, and aggressiveness.

Surgery

Surgery imposes a considerable mental threat when general anesthesia is used, and the incidence of postsurgical mental deterioration is fairly high, preventing many patients from returning to premorbid levels of mental activity. Although the symptoms are frequently transient, in almost 30 percent of geriatric surgery cases changes following general anesthesia present as confusion, loss of memory, and loss of cognitive ability. Abnormal postoperative disturbances may last from 4–5 days, but may also be present six weeks following surgery. A natural fear of going to sleep and not awakening is common in the aged, necessitating reassurance and psychological preparation prior to surgery.

Drugs also influence anesthesia management. Depressed patients may be receiving antidepressant drugs, particularly tricyclic antidepressants, which, due to their anticholinergic effect, may cause tachycardia and minor electrocardiographic changes. If the depressed patient is also hypertensive and receiving antihypertensive medication, an effect of the interaction between the two drugs may be cardiac failure. Monoamine oxidase inhibitors also influence anesthesia, since it is now known that they potentiate central nervous system depressants such as anesthetics and narcotic analgesics.

Stress

Stressors in the lives of the elderly are varied and multiple; surgery, losses of loved ones and friends, isolation and bereavement, economic insecurity, or awareness of progressive, irrevocable physical and mental decline. Stress experienced in early life may have protracted consequences that are later manifested as social and psychological sequelae. Contrary to opinion, diminished sensory acuity does not reduce receptivity to sensory bombardment but rather, like a defective hearing aid, merely scrambles sound and neural noise. Stressors of any etiology constitute a threat to the organism that demands a response. Confrontation with stress activates emotional and physiological mechanisms that enable the organism to react, but often any reaction is preempted by the nature of stress itself, and a negative state of arousal is sustained. Physiological manifestations of sustained negative arousal are evident in musculoskeletal, metabolic, endocrine, and cardiovascular changes.

The ease with which homeostasis is forfeited in the elderly is of concern here. Even minor stress will require the hypothalamus–pituitary complex to activate more hormone than is required by the young for homeostasis to be restored. Naturally lessened functional organ reserve and susceptibility to homeostatic imbalance help to explain the greater incidence of pathological disorders such as hypertension, diabetes, myocardial infarction, and atherosclerosis in the aged. The age-related lessening of central nervous system and autonomic nervous system regulatory acuity, in combination with organ decline and disease, account in part for the declines in cognitive, learning, and reactivity performance patterns. The imposition of continued subjection to stress only serves to accelerate already existing propensities toward disequilibrium. Yet, predisposition to hypertension or diabetes fails to explain the mechanisms by which stress so successfully exacerbates physical and mental dysfunction.

Hans Selye's theory of stress (1970) defined stressors as nonspecific stimuli of sufficient magnitude to disturb internal equilibrium. His general adaptation syndrome (GAS) is composed of three stages; alarm, resistance, and exhaustion. During the alarm stage confrontation with stimuli initiates a shock phase during which general systemic damage occurs, and a counter-shock phase when the organism defends itself through release of corticosteroids into the blood stream. The second stage, resistance, is characterized by a summoning of all past experience with sustained exposure to stimuli that have resulted in adaptation to stress. At this stage mobilization of all physiological resources takes place. Exhaustion, in the final stage, represents summated systemic reactions to overexposure to stress which the organism once successfully adapted to but is presently no longer able to accomplish.

The significance of GAS theory lies in the erosive acceleration of normal aging processes that result from continued exposure to stressful stimuli. Adaptation energy, like functional organ reserve, is used up so rapidly that the aged individual is increasingly unable to adapt to environmental demands. Fight or flight responses to environmental demands are mediated by perception and by either a sympathetic adrenal medullary system, or pituitary adrenal cortical response. Fight reactions arise via the hypothalamus and arousal of the adrenal medullary system with a release of the hormones norepinephrine and epinephrine, with consequent increases in cardiac output, heart rate, and blood pressure. There is some evidence from studies of biochemical precursors in laboratory animals that this fight mechanism may be decreased with age, suggesting a reduced ability to cope physiologically with stress (Selye, 1970). Flight reactions result from perception of stressors as overwhelming, or as portents of defeat, failure, or loss of control. Impulses from the hippocampal and septal regions are relayed to the anterior pituitary via the hypothalamus, activating release of ACTH and corticosteroids from the adrenal cortex. The rise in blood pressure and decrease in reticuloendothelial system function that follows suggests a greater susceptibility to infection, a phenomenon frequently observed in persons under sustained stress, and a serious consideration in the elderly. A shifting of adrenal medullary response (fight) to pituitary adrenal cortical response (flight) has been discussed by Renner and Birren (1980). Adrenal cortical response may, with age, gradually predominate over the adrenal medullary response, suggesting greater subordination rather than aggression, and a stockpiling of unexpressed emotion. Two other endocrine systems are important to this discussion. They are the ergotropic and trophotropic units, which are oppositional but reciprocal, each having CNS, ANS, and neuroendocrine components. The ergotropic unit is associated with arousal, increased activity, and elevated emotional responsivity, while the trophotropic unit is associated with diminished arousal, inactivity, and sleep. The ergotropic unit is associated with release of biogenic amines, norepinephrine and dopamine as neurotransmitters, while the trophtropic unit is associated with release of serotonin and acetylcholine. When stress is introduced and can be evaluated, an individual may confront the stimulus (ergotropic response), or avoid it (trophotropic response). Ergotropic activity is characterized by improved muscle tone, sympathetic nervous activity, and the release of catabolic hormonal products. Trophotropic inactivity is an attempt to conserve energy and permit withdrawal, and is thus characterized by decreased skeletal muscle tone, increased parasympathetic nervous function, and circulation of anabolic hormones.

Psychiatric symptoms may represent these opposing systems operating independently or simultaneously in an attempt to adapt in response to stress. Acute fearfulness may result from dominance of the trophotropic unit, while chronic tension may be the result of ergotropic dominance. Simultaneous discharge of the two systems may result in anxiety, agitated depression, delirium, or acute schizophreniform psychotic disintegration. The latter may occur without loss of consciousness or memory, and may be manifested by hallucinations, delusions, or thought disorders. Such symptoms may appear in any age group, but because of the increased propensity for cerebral inefficiency, the elderly are considerably more prone to delirium-like manifestations resulting from stress.

SUMMARY

This chapter has focused on examples of neuropsychiatric symptomtology that emanate from underlying physiological disorders. Confusion, one of the most common symptoms in old age, has been a result of almost every disorder discussed. It has been shown to result from cerebral embolization, cardiac conduction defects, and antihypertensive agents, to name but a few. Renal system impairment may present as lethargy, acute psychosis, irritability or depression. Impaired judgment, apprehension, combativeness, and disorientation have all been associated with chronic and acute respiratory disease.

Confusional episodes may be the only presenting symptom of chronic hepatitis, just as depression may be the only presenting symptom of cancer of the pancreas. Vitamins play a significant role in geriatric mental health and vitamin deficiencies involving iron, B_{12}, and folate, may exhibit symptoms of dementia, disorientation, and depression, all in the absence of anemia. Hypothyroidism as the source of classical "dementia" is examined in conjunction with other subtle changes in endocrine function. Changes in the central nervous system have been shown to effect neurological, psychological, and emotional functions in highly diverse ways.

Intellectual, cognitive, and emotional functions are all subject to the subtle influences of disease interacting with age-related physiological change, with these functions in turn being influenced by drugs, trauma, and stress. The biochemical effects of altered neurotransmitters, CNS receptivity, and drug toxicity, are discussed as potentially high risk factors in surgery for the elderly. Stress is examined from the theoretical perspective of general adaptation syndrome, and a stimuli to ergotropic or trophotropic units operating in opposition or reciprocity to each other in the establishment and maintenance of homeostasis.

REFERENCES

Altman, H., Mehta, D., Evenson, R., & Sletten, I. (1973). Behavioral effects of drug therapy on psychogeriatric patients. II. Multivitamin supplement. *Journal of the American Geriatrics Society, 21,* 249–252.

Anderson, W. F. (1966). The prevention of illness in the elderly: The Rutherglen experiment in medicine in old age. *Proceedings of the Royal College of Physicians.* London: Pittman.

Cogan, M., Covey, C., Arieff, A., et al. (1978). Central nervous system manifestations of hyperparathyroidism. *American Journal of Medicine, 65,* 963–970.

Drachman, D. (1980). An approach to the neurology of aging. In J. Birren & R. Sloane (Eds.), *Handbook of mental health and aging* (pp. 501–519). Englewood Cliffs, NJ: Prentice-Hall.

Fields, W. (1981). Psychiatric manifestations of central nervous system disorders. In A. Levenson & R. Hall (Eds.), *Neuropsychiatric manifestations of physical disease in the elderly. Aging series,* vol. 14 (pp. 17–27). New York: Raven Press.

Gershell, W. (1981). Psychiatric manifestations and nutritional deficiencies in the elderly. In A. Levenson & R. Hall (Eds.), *Neuropsychiatric manifestations of physical disease in the elderly. Aging series, vol. 14* (pp. 119–131). New York: Raven Press.

Hall, W. (1981). Psychiatric problems in the elderly related to organic pulmonary disease. In A. Levenson & R. Hall (Eds.), *Neuropsychiatric manifestations of physical disease in the elderly. Aging series, vol. 14* (pp. 41–48). New York: Raven Press.

Hall, R., Levenson, A., & LeCann, A. (1981). Evaluation and assessment of nonfunctional psychiatric illness in the elderly. In A. Levensen & R. Hall (Eds.), *Neuropsychiatric manifestations of physical disease in the elderly. Aging series, vol. 14* (pp. 133–149). New York: Raven Press.

Hoffman, N. (1981). Gastrointestinal diseases presenting as psychiatric symptoms. In A. Levenson & R. Hall (Eds.), *Neuropsychiatric manifestations of physical disease in the elderly. Aging series, Vol. 14* (pp. 49-57). New York: Raven Press.

Karpati, G., & Frame, B. (1964). Neuropsychiatric disorders in primary hyperpara-thyroidism. *Archives of Neurology, 10,* 387-397.

Kinsman, R., & Hood, H. (1971). Some behavioral effects of ascorbic acid deficiency. *American Journal of Clinical Nutrition, 24:* 455–464.

Lavis, V. (1981). Psychiatric manifestations of endocrine disease in the elderly. In A. Levenson & R. Hall (Eds.), *Neuropsychiatric manifestations of physical disease in the elderly. Aging series, Vol. 14* (pp. 59–81). New York: Raven Press.

Libow, L. (1973). Pseudosenility: Acute and reversible organic brain syndrome. *Journal of the American Geriatrics Society, 21,* 112–120.

Minaker, K., & Rowe, J. (1981). Behavioral manifestations of renal disease in the elderly. In A. Levenson & R. Hall (Eds.), *Neuropsychiatric manifestations of physical disease in the elderly. Aging series, Vol. 14* (93–102). New York: Raven Press.

Renner, V. & Birren, J. (1980). Stress: Physiological and psychological mechanisms. In J. Birren & R. Sloane (Eds.), *Handbook of mental health and aging* (pp. 310–336). Englewood Cliffs, NJ: Prentice-Hall, Inc.

Rosenberg, G. (1981). Neuropsychiatric manifestations of cardiovascular disease in the elderly. In A. Levenson & R. Hall (Eds.), *Neuropsychiatric manifestations of Physical Disease in the Elderly. Aging Series, vol. 14.* (pp. 29–39). New York: Raven Press.

Selye, H. (1970). Stress and aging. Journal of the American Geriatrics Society, 18, 669–680.

United States Senate (1976). Special Committee on Aging, Subcommittee on Long-Term Care and on Health of the Elderly. *Joint hearings: Medicare and medicaid frauds.* Washington, DC: U.S. Government Printing Office.

Weinger, R. (1981). Psychiatric manifestations of hematopoietic system disease. In A. Levenson & R. Hall (Eds.), *Neuropsychiatric manifestations of physical disease in the elderly. Aging series, vol. 14* (pp. 83–92). New York: Raven Press.

SUGGESTED READINGS

Corriere, J. (1981). Psychiatric manifestations of lower urinary tract disease in the elderly. In A. Levenson & R. Hall (Eds.), *Neuropsychiatric manifestations of physical disease in the elderly. Aging series, vol. 14* (pp. 103–109). New York: Raven Press.

Grob, D. (1978). Common disorders of muscles in the aged. In W. Reichel (Ed.), *Clinical aspects of aging* (pp. 245–259). Baltimore: Williams and Wilkins Co.

Habot, B. & Libow, L. (1980). The interrelationship of mental and physical status and its assessment in the older adult: Mind–Body interaction. In J. Birren & R. Sloane (Eds.), *Handbook of mental health and aging* (pp. 701–716). Englewood Cliffs, NJ: Prentice-Hall Inc.

Lindeman, R. (1978). Application of fluid and electrolyte balance principles to the older patient. In W. Reichel (Ed.), *Clinical aspects of aging* (pp. 213–226). Baltimore: Williams and Wilkins Co.

Locke, S., & Galaburda, A. (1978). Neurological disorders of the elderly. In W. Reichel (Ed.), *Clinical aspects of aging* (pp. 133–138). Baltimore: Williams and Wilkins Co.

Spencer, H., & Lender, M. (1979). The skeletal system. In I. Rossman (Ed.), *Clinical geriatrics,* 2nd ed (pp. 460–476). Philadelphia: Lippincott Co.

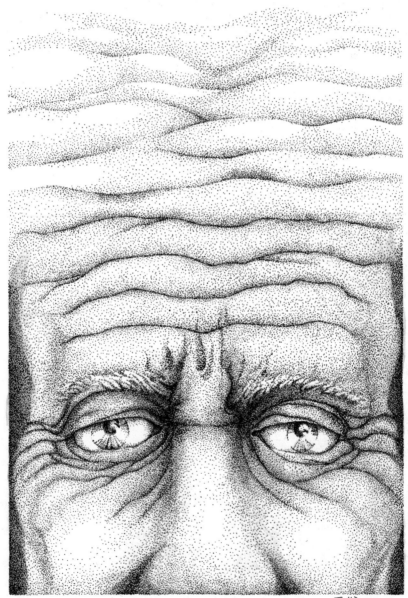

Tull-Bowers

94

Chapter 7

Assessment and Differentiation

As the numbers of elderly patients increase, bringing into the health care system complexities of systemic and neuropsychiatric interaction, the demands made upon health professionals increase proportionately. Already burdened by excessive workloads, they struggle to meet these increased demands, and in the vast majority of cases do so successfully.

Occasionally, however, diagnostic errors, iatrogenic illnesses, and imprecise evaluations occur. Terminological inconsistencies, masking effects, fluctuations in symptomatology, and limitations of present knowledge, all contribute to inaccurate estimations. Three problem areas, confusion, depression, and psychosis, all frequently encountered in care of the aged patient, are addressed in this chapter in order to strengthen the clinician's skill at differential assessment.

DIAGNOSTIC ERRORS

Accurate diagnosis of brain disorders of elderly subjects is difficult, due in part to the previously stated fact that morphologic changes may not always be sufficient to account for dementia, and may be found in the absence of dementia. The diagnostic problem is also hindered by what Wells (1978) describes as the inescapable conclusion that diagnostic errors, both of omission and commission, may result from both organic (senile) and functional (affective) disorders. For example, physicians may fail to recognize cerebral disease when it is present to a significant degree because they fail to ask the significant questions; asking the questions rather than assuming the answers is essential, because patients with dementia seldom complain of its characteristic symptoms, but will often report other somatic or affectual discomforts that suggest other diagnoses. Often only family members or close friends can provide a correct perspective, but they are not always consulted. Error might arise from the misdiagnosis of dementia when in fact the patient has pseudodementia. Here the diagnostic errors result from failure to heed sufficiently the patient's behavior, which frequently suggests a level of brain function inconsistent with the severity of dysfunction suggested by mental status examination.

Gaitz (1982) suggests that the multifaceted problems of the elderly patient present diagnostic difficulties by requiring broad rather than narrowly defined diagnoses. The findings of a broad diagnostic approach may raise questions about etiology and the relative importance of certain findings, while the traditionally narrow approach is less likely to generate uncertainty. Reliance upon physical examination and test results to the exclusion of social and psychological factors has been common. Diagnosticians who strive for precision and specificity as routes to specific interventions and effective treatment sometimes challenge multiple diagnoses as imprecise and inaccurate. Training has traditionally emphasized as few diagnoses as possible, with explanations related to a single diagnosis if possible. Reality, however, is that most elderly patients, when carefully examined, are found to have several disorders presenting simultaneously and producing interacting physical and mental symptoms. Because of this the likelihood of diagnostic errors is increased. Schouten (1975) reports two instances of diagnostic error:

> Two elderly ward patients were diagnosed as "mentally confused" and because of their mental state were to be transferred to a psychogeriatric unit. Clinical and laboratory data revealed that both had sustained heart attacks. Upon treatment and recovery, symptoms of mental confusion disappeared.

> Another patient who was diagnosed as demented, was cured of mental symptoms by having his ear canals syringed. Failing to hear what was being said to him, he did not respond appropriately to questions, and was assumed to be senile.

Sloane (1980) reports that approximately 40 percent of chronically hospitalized psychiatric patients suffer primarily from "unrecognized" physical brain disorders. He cites two studies:

> In one investigation 80 randomly picked patients suffering from "organic brain syndrome" in a VA hospital, were actually found to have a wide range of diagnoses.

> In another investigation, of 106 patients admitted with presumptive diagnosis of dementia, only 84 were conclusively demonstrated to be so. Of 15 patients found to be suffering from other illnesses, depression was found most commonly, followed by drug toxicity.

IATROGENIC DISORDERS

Iatrogenic disorders, or those induced by care givers or health system processes also accentuate the need for diagnostic accuracy. Drug-induced complications and diseases are most often implicated, and Butler (1979) cites two examples:

Acute brain disorders have been created by the use of over-prescribed tranquilizers for elderly patients.

Uncontrolled use of phenothiazines—Thorazine or Mellaril—frequently results in tardive dyskinesia whose irreversible manifestations may become evident only after withdrawal of the offending drug.

The need to prevent diagnostic errors and iatrogenic illnesses should obviously remain uppermost in the minds of health care professionals as they undertake assessment and treatment interventions. To that end, this chapter focuses on three more ambiguous areas in geriatric mental health; confusion, depression and psychosis.

ASSESSMENT AND DIFFERENTIATION

Differential diagnosis is difficult under the best of circumstances, and particularly so with the older patient who presents a multiplicity of symptoms and neuropsychiatric manifestations of varied physical diseases. Patients and professionals alike labor to overcome mental illnesses that yield diverse clinical symptomatology and lack precise terminology. As a result, the etiological classifications of illnesses presenting as "dementia" tend to be only approximate. Sloane (1980) estimates that despite comprehensive investigation, a definite diagnosis can be reached only in about 50 percent of all demented patients. Terminological imprecision is most evident in references to "confusion" and "confusional states" which, far from being disease states, reflect transitional evidence of cerebral dysfunction. The symptoms suggest alterations in mentation, orientation, and behavior. Table 7-1 lists common factors which affect mentation and result in somewhat different behavior patterns for functionally and organically confused persons. Symptoms cited for organic confusion refer to findings common for dementia, rather than the more florid fluctuations of delirium.

ASSESSMENT OF CONFUSION

Despite the frequency with which the word confusion is used, few commonly agreed upon definitions have been proposed, and considerable subjectivity still exists. Plum and Posner (1972) describe confusion as a

Table 7-1 Differential Assessment of Functional and Organic Confusion

Factor	Functional	Organic
Ideation	Complex and Varied	Simple and slowed
Language	Appropriate to bizarre	Neologisms and tangential responses common
Learning capacity	Usually good	Poor
Memory	May be faulty but usually good	Recent memory poor—confuses past and present
Abstract thought	Varied	Impaired
Intellect	Flexible responses	Stimulus-bound response
Insight	Usually good	Usually poor
Judgment	Varied	Poor
Consciousness	Usually unimpaired	Preoccupation progresses to stupor
Unresponsiveness	Uncommon	Common
Orientation		
Time	Good to aberrant	Deteriorated
Place	Bizarre	Confuses familiar with unfamiliar; deteriorates
Person	Not usually preserved	Usually preserved
Perception of others	Misidentifies delusional content	Misidentifies known, familiar persons
Anxiety	Varied	Catastrophic reaction
Hallucinations	Auditory, bizarre, symbolic	Rare
Delusions	Bizarre, symbolic	Mudane, paranoid
Illusions	Not prominent	Prominent; misperception of sensory data
Periodicity	Consistency	Inconsistency
Nocturnal		
wandering	Uncommon	Common
Incontinence	Continent	Incontinent

manifestation of clouded consciousness that includes disorientation, sensory misperception, and alternating periods of excitability and drowsiness. The patient is startled by minor stimuli, easily distracted, unable to think clearly or quickly, and consistently misinterprets stimuli. Attention span is shortened, the patient is bewildered, and often has difficulty following commands. Memory is faulty and diurinal drowsiness often alternates with nocturnal agitation. The clinical features described by Plum and Posner include the following.

Alertness. Altered awareness is the first and most subtle index of brain dysfunction. Initial disinterest or preoccupation progresses to lethargy and stupor.

Orientation and Grasp. Defects in orientation and immediate grasp of test situations are often the earliest unequivocal symptoms of brain dysfunction. Demented patients tend to lose orientation and cognition long before lethargy develops.

Cognition and Attention. The content and progression of thought are always disturbed in delirium and dementia, sometimes presenting as the incipient symptoms.

Memory. Loss of recent memory is a hallmark of dementia, and is frequent in delirium. Memory loss and an inability to form new associations can be a sign of either diffuse or bilateral focal brain disease.

Affect. Apathetic withdrawal is common, but agitated responses may also alternate with apathy.

Perception. Perceptual errors and illusory mistakes are common (e.g., bedside rails appear to be jailhouse bars, cardiac monitors resemble TV screens).

The differential diagnosis of organic and psychogenic unresponsiveness of conscious patients includes differences in mental state, EEG, motor signs, and occasionally breathing patterns. Conscious organically dysfunctional patients are confused and disoriented, abstract thinking is defective, concentration is poor, and new information is not easily retained. During early stages, their outstretched dorsiflexed hands show irregular tremulousness, and frequently asterixis. Snouting, sucking, and grasping reflexes are seen. EEG is generally slow. Hypo- or hyperventilation may occur, as well as posthyperventilation apnea. In contrast, conscious psychogenic patients are rarely disoriented, and are able to use new information. Abnormal reflexes or adventitious movements are absent, and EEG frequencies are normal. Ventilatory patterns are usually normal. While unresponsiveness is common among organic patients, psychogenic unresponsiveness sustained for more than a few minutes is uncommon.

Brocklehurst (1975) recommends a step-by-step approach to the assessment of confusion, and suggests the following sequence:

1. A detailed history of the complaint with special reference to:
    rate of evolution of the mental disturbance
    evidence of failing intellectual or social capacity
    drug therapy
    major social unheavals
    coexistent physical symptoms
    previous hospital admissions and reasons
    known history of prior mental disorder
    patient's pre-morbid personality
    mood changes

2. Physical examination and observation of behavior
3. Ancillary investigations for detection of occult physical disease
4. Psychometric assessment

Precursive Conditions

Precursive conditions that facilitate the onset of confusional symptoms in the aged patient include:

- Physiological changes in organs and organ systems
- Language and cultural differences
- Neurosensory deficits (hearing, vision, touch, etc.)
- Unavailable prostheses (eyeglasses, dentures, hearing aids, artificial limbs, etc.)
- Neural noise interference with normal message transmission
- Drugs
- Environmental disruption (hospital relocation, confinement, loss of normal routine, restraints, etc.)
- Environmental distortion (distortion of light, dark, time, space, sleeping cycles, etc.)
- Sensory Imbalance (sensory deprivation, isolation, overload)
- Decision or time demands that conflict with environmental expectations
- Rapid fluctuating change

Each of the conditions mentioned is brought to bear during the admission of any older patient into hospitals, so it is hardly remarkable that the incidence of confusion is so very high.

Two additional factors further complicate the problem. Gotestam (1980) and several others (Feinberg, 1975; Sloane, 1980) subsequently have shown that confused, disorganized behavior could be produced during the day if a patient was placed in a darkened room, lending support to the notion that confusion is a function of the level of background stimulation. The effect of stereotype on perceptions of confusion is equally disturbing. Chisholm, Deniston, Igrisan, & Barbus (1982) recently showed that a self-fulfilling prophecy effect can take place insidiously within the hospital ward. The findings revealed that if a ''confused'' patient was to be segregated from ''non-confused'' patients, segregation practices of the staff correlated positively with their definitions of confusion. In effect, some non-confused patients became grouped by association with the stereotypically confused. An additional finding, one that certainly warrants further investigation, was the lack of confusion at the time of admission or soon thereafter: less than ten percent of the patients exhibited symptoms of confusion on admission or within the first 24 hours. Clearly the impact of environment and attitude seem to be influencing the ways in which confusion is perceived and dealt with in in-patient settings.

ASSESSMENT OF DEPRESSION

Due to the fact that depression may mimic dementia, and often coexists with dementia in the early stages of brain dysfunction, differential assessment of the two conditions is strongly recommended. The depressive symptoms that are common especially early in dementia diminish as it progresses. Memory deficit is apparent initially, accompanied by apathy, lack of spontaneity, and a quiet withdrawal from social interactions. Confirmation of a differential diagnosis will often necessitate a follow-up by longitudinal observations, since longterm outcomes of treatment will differ. Table 7-2 presents prevalent, characteristic symptoms of unipolar depression and dementia in the aged, that should be evaluated as part of the assessment process.

Certain areas of mental functioning, such as learning and orientation, are thought to aid in the task of assessment. The preservation of orientation and learning are thought to distinguish the functional depressive from patients in the first stages of degenerative brain diseases. According to Folstein and McHugh (1978) patients diagnosed as organically impaired with depressive features are only rarely disoriented, and their learning abilities are not completely lost. Elderly depressed patients also show clear depressive symptoms and a frequent history of affective attacks. The differential diagnosis rests on these clinical features and the paucity of neurological signs and laboratory evidence of brain disease, such as aphasia or lateralizing deficits.

A complete history is imperative in order to place any depressive episodes within the context of the patient's life history. Have episodes occurred before, and if so, how were they treated? Of particular importance is the determination of whether the patient has a history of repeated similar episodes or whether a present episode is to be interpreted as a response to increasing organic deficit. Freedman, Kaplan, & Sadock (1976) believe that late-onset depressives, in comparison with early-onset patients, have better adjusted personalities emotionally, socially, and psychosexually. The majority of first, late-onset attacks usually follow closely the occurrence of some traumatic event—bereavement, loss of job or status, or the threat of physical illness. The history is also important in terms of a rather salient point that Freden (1982) makes in regard to the aged patient. The older we become, the more likely we are to be forced to leave the shelter of familiar, established walls. Even more important, we have become more firmly enmeshed in a fixed conceptual world, one that becomes more limited, and one that limits our actions to settled routines that are difficult to alter. Older

Table 7-2 Differential Assessment of Depression and Dementia

Factors	Depression	Dementia
Onset	Abrupt	Gradual, insidious
Periodicity	Little variation	Symptoms worsen at night—Sundowner's Syndrome
Somatic symptoms	Anorexia, weight loss, psychomotor retardation may mimic dementia	Progressive psychomotor loss
Neurologic exam	Negative	Positive
Intellect	Mild to moderate performance loss may mimic demetia	Impaired
Cognition	Intact but may mimic loss	Impaired
Learning capacity	Usually retained	Impaired
Spatial perception	Unchanged	Impaired
Orientation	Well oriented	Disoriented
Judgment	Intact	Impaired
Abstract thought	Intact	Impaired
Memory	Unimpaired but may mimic loss	Progressive loss
Speech	Slowed response	Often aphasic
Affect	Deeper depressive troughs, consistent depression, irritability, hostility	Shallow mood change, inconsistent or episodic depression Shallowness, catastrophic anxiety
Delusions	Uncommon	Common
Hallucinations	Uncommon	Common
Appearance	Disinterest	Habit deterioration
Behavior	Withdrawal, tearful, hypochondriacal	Given to outbursts
Sleep	Insomnia, early morning awakening	Impaired, restless, fitful
Suicidal ideation	Positive	Negative
EEG	Unchanged	Slow-wave activity increased
History of recent stress	Positive, precipitating event	Negative
Response to treatment	Dramatic improvement	Little change
Continence	Continent	Incontinent
Prognosis	Good	Poor

patients frequently perceive interventions such as the assessment interview and history as intrusions into their personal and psychological domain; invasions that may be potentially beneficial, but are immediately threatening. Cognitive, neurosensory, or even social deficits, if publicly identified, bode even more intrusion and disruption of personal lifestyle. Because of this, deficits will often be denied or dismissed as inconsequential. The patient's social supports, be they family or friends, may also conceal cognitive deficits, particularly if they have been intervening in such activities as grocery shopping or making appointments. For this reason it is important to explore well beyond the routine checks of memory or orientation. In addition to asking "Where are you?" and "What day is it?" ask how the patient manages his own finances, balances a checkbook, or makes and keeps his own medical appointments.

ASSESSMENT OF PSYCHOSIS

Because of the unknown etiology of functional and organic disorders, and the unknown relationship between cause and symptoms, Feinberg (1975) indicates that the classification of psychiatric disorders must be symptomatic. Psychoses as a classificatory category refers to symptoms that suggest a distortion of reality due to impaired thinking or feeling (functional psychosis), or to grossly impaired consciousness and information processing (organic psychosis). Some distinctions exist, however, between the two categories, and these aid in differential diagnosis.

In functional disorders the sensorium is generally intact, but functionally disordered persons will make errors on tests of sensorium that are qualitatively different from those made by organically disordered persons. Functional disorders exhibit mood, behavior, and thought disturbances that often reflect specific psychiatric meanings and motivations.

In organic disorders, sensorium is impaired, and characteristic behaviors are produced that are not historically expected and, as Hall, Levenson, & Le Cann (1981) suggest, are stimulus-bound and fragmented.

Both types of disorders may coexist in old age, but must be considered separately because of differing diagnostic techniques and intervention requirements. Outcomes differ as well, with a favorable prognosis for functional illness and an extremely poor prognosis for organic illness. An additional concern, strongly supportive of differential diagnosis, is that neurological abnormalities are more prevalent among psychiatric populations than is ordinarily suspected. Small (1973) suggests that much psychiatric disturbance may be intensified by or attributable to brain dysfunction, a position that clearly argues for early differential diagnosis and treatment.

Although the clinical picture witnessed by practitioners rarely if ever coincides with textbook descriptions, and coexistent symptoms in the older patient will allow "classical" syndromes with even greater rarity, the more characteristic symptoms of functional and organic psychosis are presented in Table 7-3. The findings are summarized into highly oversimplified categories to assist in depicting normative distinctions between the two populations. Deviations according to subcategories will cloud the assessment picture, and it must be remembered that coexistent functional psychosis and even mild brain damage will defy differential diagnoses.

Several points should be made about areas of commonality and difference in both types of disorder. Supporting commonality, Cath (1976) believes that functional illness related to stress always has an organic or biochemical substrate that, at any age, may trigger a disorder of metabolic importance such that in time healthy tissue is converted into areas of nondemonstrable but still pathological foci. Further, human responses to organic deficit—an observing, despairing ego that mourns the loss of normal bodily functioning—present as an active part of the overall clinical picture, and must be included in the behavioral assessment.

Supporting difference between the two types of disorder are characteristic findings regarding illness onset and course. Senile psychosis is most often a slow passage, from normal old age to psychosis, that Butler (1979) describes as free of any marked or abrupt change. It differs also from paraphrenic illnesses, which tend similarly to be chronic, but are not characterized by the severe deterioration of personality and habits.

Neuropsychological Assessments

Neuropsychological assessments are proving to be increasingly useful in discriminating organic from functional disorders. An impressive body of evidence documents that organic disorders show a wide range of neuropsychological disturbances, while functional disorders do not. Miller (1981) indicates that organic patients are frequently unable to answer orientation questions and will reveal particular impairment on tests of spatial perception and praxis, and errors and delays in naming on tests of speech. Memory impairment as well is much less severe in functional psychosis than it is in organic illness. Malignant memory loss is considered typical of organic disease, as an indicant of severely impaired recall and recognition capacities. Repeated presentations of the same test paragraph to functional and organic patients yield different results; those suffering from functional illnesses perform well, gaining recall and recognition benefits which accumulate with each presentation, while those suffering from organic illness do not.

Psychological testing makes an invaluable contribution to the diagnostic armamentarium. Poor performance on the Wechsler Adult Intelligence Scale (W.A.I.S.) subtests (particularly information and comprehension) may be indicative of senile psychosis. If standardized psychological tests are

Table 7-3 Differential Assessment of Functional and Organic Psychosis

Factors	Functional (affective)	Organic (senile)
Onset	Usually abrupt	Gradual, insidious
Course	Self-limiting, recurrance	Steady, progressive deterioration
Appearance	Disinterest	Dilapidation, excrement carelessness
Behavior	Hyper- or hypoactive, motivational	Initially unremarkable, later given to outbursts and wandering, stimulus-bound and fragmented
Intellect	Unimpaired	Marked impairment
Attention, concentration	Fair to good	Poor
Abstract thought	Abstraction good	Abstraction poor, concrete
Comprehension, coherence	Good	Very poor
Learning ability	Fair to good	Very poor
Memory	Fair to good, may be well preserved	Marked impairment, very poor recall-recognition
Judgment	Fair to good	Poor, errors
Insight	Fair to good	Absent
Sensorium	Intact, well oriented	Marked disorientation
Confusional states	Not prominent	Gross, worse at night, transitory fearfulness
Perception		
Illusions	Rare	Common
Hallucinations	Rare, but auditory possible	Episodic auditory, worse at night
Delusions	Consistent with affect state	Persistent paranoid tendencies
Affect, mood	Elation, depression	Emotional lability, emotional incontinence, superficial depression related to anxiety
Speech	Slowed	Dysphasic, rambling, incoherent, errors and delays in naming
Psychomotor function	Retardation, agitation	Tremors, muscle rigidity, poor visual-motor coordination
Personality	Temporary regression	Loosened inhibitions, severe habit deterioration
Neurologic exam	Negative	Positive
EEG	Unchanged	Increased slow-wave activity
Response to treatment	Favorable to drugs and ECT	Poor
Continence	Continent	Incontinent
Prognosis	Good	Very poor

administered slowly, they will demonstrate the presence or absence of organic impairment, and whether the disorder results in an inability to produce answers or to formulate them. Repeated testing (serially) is also recommended, since this may unequivocally demonstrate the progression of intellectual loss necessary for adequate diagnosis.

SUMMARY

Diagnostic errors and iatrogenic illnesses are unacceptable on professional, moral, and ethical grounds, and accentuate the need for accuracy in mental status assessment. Traditional practices such as seeking a single diagnosis in pursuit of diagnostic accuracy must be replaced with cognizance of many causative factors that coexist and alter the aged patient's mental status. Confusion, a frequent concomitant of underlying pathophysiological processes, is examined as a manifestation of organic and functional illness. Differences in responsiveness, orientation, memory, consciousness, and periodicity help to differentiate confusion of functional from organic etiology. Environment and attitude may play an instrumental role in the ways in which confusion is perceived by both patient and staff, and the ways in which those perceptions effect treatment regimen.

Depression often mimics dementia, and a differential assessment should highlight differences in cognitive functions such as learning ability, judgment, abstraction, spatial perception, orientation, affect, delusion, and hallucination. Differences in onset, response to treatment, and prognosis are also apparent.

Functional and organic psychosis have been discussed, with differences in sensorium, onset, illness course, memory, and perception indicated. Memory and sensorium play pivotal roles in differential diagnosis. Neuropsychological assessment is increasingly valuable in identifying organically related deficits and the deteriorative trajectory of brain dysfunction in the elderly.

REFERENCES

Brocklehurst, J. (1975). *Geriatric medicine for students*. Edinburgh: Churchill Livingstone. 1976.

Butler, R. (1979). Psychiatry. In I. Rossman (Ed.), *Clinical geriatrics* (pp. 519–550). Philadelphia: J.B. Lippincott.

Cath, S. (1976). Functional disorders: An organismic view and attempt at reclassification. In L. Bellak & T. Karasu (Eds.), *Geriatric psychiatry* (pp. 141–172). New York: Grune & Stratton, Inc.

Chisholm, S., Deniston, O., Igrisan, R., & Barbus, A. (1982). Prevalence of confusion in elderly hospitalized patients. Journal of Gerontology Nursing, *8*(2), 87–96.

Feinberg, I. (1975). The psychiatric work-up. In I. Glick (Ed.), *Syllabus—introduction to clinical psychiatry* (pp. 5–18). San Francisco: University of California.

Folstein, M., & McHugh P. (1978). Dementia syndrome of depression. In R. Katzman, R. Terry, & K. Bick (Eds.), *Alzheimer's disease: Senile dementia and related disorders. Aging series, Vol. 7* (pp. 87–93). New York: Raven Press.

Freden, L. (1982). *Psychosocial aspects of depression.* New York: John Wiley and Sons.

Freedman, A., Kaplan, H., & Sadock, B. (1976). *Modern synopsis of comprehensive textbook of psychiatry II.* Baltimore: Williams and Wilkins Co.

Gaitz, C. (1982). Some psychophysiological problems of the elderly. In W. Fann, I. Karacan, A. Pokorny, & R. Williams (Eds.), *Phenomenology and treatment of psychophysiological disorders* (pp. 191–202). New York: Spectrum Publications, Inc.

Gotestam, K. (1980) Behavioral and dynamic psychotherapy with the elderly. In J. Birren & R. Sloane (Eds.), *Handbook of mental health and aging* (pp. 775–805). Englewood Cliffs, NJ: Prentice-Hall, Inc.

Hall, R., Levenson, A., & LeCann, A. (1981). Evaluation and assessment of nonfunctional psychiatric illness in the elderly. In A. Levenson & R. Hall (Eds.), *Neuropsychiatric manifestations of physical disease in the elderly. Aging Series, vol. 14* (pp. 133–149). New York: Raven Press. 149.

Miller, E. (1981). The differential psychological evaluation. In N. Miller & G. Cohen (Eds.), *Clinical aspects of Alzheimer's disease and senile dementia. Aging Series, vol. 15* (pp. 121–138). New York: Raven Press.

Plum, F. & Posner, J. (1972). *The diagnosis of stupor and coma.* Philadelphia: F.A. Davis Company.

Schouten, J. (1975). Important factors in the examination and care of old patients. *Journal of the American Geriatrics Society, 23,* 180–183.

Sloane, R. (1980). Organic brain syndrome. In J. Birren & R. Sloane (Eds.), *Handbook of mental health and aging* (pp. 554–590). Englewood Cliffs, NJ: Prentice-Hall, Inc.

Small, L. (1973). *Neuropsychodiagnosis in psychotherapy.* New York: Brunner/Mazel.

Wells, C. (1978). Chronic brain disease: An overview. *American Journal of Psychiatry, 135* (1), 1–12.

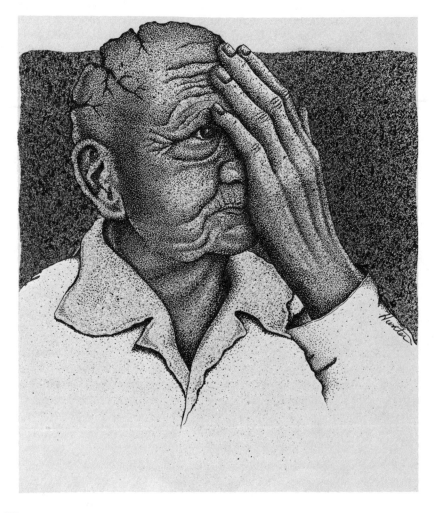

108

Chapter 8

Assessment of Organic Mental Syndrome

Assessment of organic mental syndrome is of sufficient importance to warrant special attention for several reasons. Stereotypical assumptions, reliance upon traditional single-diagnosis strategies, and use of the presently available clinical and psychometric measures as the only procedures in evaluation of dementia, have often resulted in false-positive or false-negative diagnoses. Characteristic memory and cognitive impairment may be present in the absence of verified brain impairment, while in other instances significant brain impairment may exist without marked memory or cognitive loss. Cautionary notes are being voiced from any number of disciplines about the inherent dangers of assuming that the patient who behaves in a demented fashion is indeed suffering from chronic organic brain syndrome. A false-positive diagnosis derives from the stereotype of the inevitability of senility in the aged which, in combination with poor physical health, cultural deficits, and depressed affect, may lead to inappropriate treatment and negligent deterioration. A false-negative diagnosis, seen most often in the patient with acute organic mental syndrome, denies opportunities for reversing that which is still reversible, and sentences the patient to progressive deterioration. This chapter examines the similarities and differences of both acute and chronic disorders as manifested by prominent features, clinical signs and stages, and key concepts.

ASSESSMENT OF ACUTE ORGANIC MENTAL SYNDROME

Assessment of the syndrome requires a thorough historical, physical, neurological, and mental status examination. Sloane (1980) recommends that a complete history, taken from a reliable informant, focus on the identification of recent physical illnesses, medications, and nonprescription drugs.

General physical examination should look for evidence of trauma, systemic illness, and consider the state of respiratory ventilation. The presence of focal weakness or abnormal movements is considered highly significant.

Etiology

Delirium may be caused by a wide variety of diseases or agents, all sufficient to induce characteristic changes in mentation and behavior. Structural brain disease (tumors, subdural hematomas, cerebral infarctions), functional brain disease (schizophrenia, manic–depressive psychosis), and metabolic diseases must all be considered likely etiologic agents. In addition, medications, metabolic imbalance, depression, acute emotional state, nutritional deficiencies, neuropathology, gastrointestinal, hepatic, cardiovascular, febrile, or pulmonary disorders, and surgery or trauma, may all induce the transient, reversible behaviors associated with temporary cerebral insufficiency (see Chapter 6).

Differential diagnosis is hindered by the absence of focal signs that are characteristic of young patients. Signs of intracranial tumors may be slow to develop because of the enlarged intracranial space that results from cerebral atrophy. Subdural hematoma may present insidiously, with the patient becoming merely increasingly drowsy over a period of days, then slipping into irreversible coma. Uremia, pulmonary disease or anoxia may present with a quiet, apathetic withdrawal, while alcohol or barbituate withdrawal, or hepatic necrosis, may result in agitated delirium. Dehydration, constipation, and avitaminosis are also frequently implicated in confusional episodes. Because of the diversity of etiological agents, the difference between clinical manifestations of delirium in young and old patients, and characteristic fulminant fluctuations in symptoms, the prominent features of organic brain syndrome are summarized below.

Prominent Features of Acute Organic Mental Syndrome

History

Onset of the disease is rapid, usually completed within hours or days. There is evidence of recent physical illness, and evidence of recent change in drug or alcohol intake.

Behavior

There is marked fluctuation in arousal and awareness, disorientation to time and place, and reduced attention span. Patients are easily distracted. Their state of consciousness changes rapidly; they seem bewildered, perplexed, and unable to comprehend. Thought processes are incoherent and concretized. Immediate and recent memory is poor. Hallucinations (visual, vivid, with animals, insects, colored forms) are common, particularly at night. Auditory hallucinations are also frequent. Delusions are transient, fragmented, and unsystematized. Paranoid misinterpretations are common, as are illusions, the result of over-responding to multiple extraneous stimuli. Endogenous sensory input (e.g., tinnitus) commonly causes misinterpretation of exogenous stimuli. Sleep is reduced and fitful, and mood states alternate from dreamlike trance to anxiety, and even severe terror. Restlessness, confused "searching," and "miming" of familiar activities (e.g., rocking a baby, or telling the rosary) are common.

Neurologic Signs

The presence of focal weakness and abnormal movement should be noted.

Asterixis. "Flapping tremor" (jerking movements elicited by dorsaflexion of the wrists and extension of the fingers) is seen only in delirium; it may also affect the feet and tongue and must be distinguished from tardive dyskinesia. Ask the obtunded patient to squeeze two of the examiners fingers; with asterixis the examiner can feel the patient's fingers alternately clenching and unclenching.

Multifocal Myoclonus. This is sudden, involuntary, gross muscle contractions, most common in the face and jaw of the resting patient.

Seizures, Weakness, and Hyperactive Stretch Reflexes. These are often concomitants of metabolic brain disease.

Pupillary Light Reactions. These are preserved in metabolic coma, and their absence suggests structural lesion. Fixed dilated pupils may be caused by anticholinergic drugs.

EEG. A nonspecific, bilateral symmetrical slowing, with slower activity as patient loses awareness, may be indicative acute organic brain syndrome.

Key Concepts Regarding Acute Organic Mental Syndrome

The following is a list of important concepts to be kept in mind during the assessment process.

- Acute onset often points to metabolic or drug etiology.
- The more rapid the onset of the illness, the greater the likelihood of agitation.
- A single cause is rare in the aged patient.
- Symptoms worsen at night.
- Defects in comprehension and grasp are common.

- Characteristic episodic intervals of confusion and lucidity differentiate delirium from dementia.
- Response to treatment is usually favorable.
- Acute organic mental syndrome, if untreated, may progress to chronic organic mental disease.
- When treated, full recovery is usually possible.

ASSESSMENT OF CHRONIC ORGANIC MENTAL SYNDROME

Recent or abrupt changes in mental status are not indicative of chronic mental syndrome. Etiology remains unknown, but is believed to involve some combination of neuronal loss, cortical atrophy, and arteriosclerotic disease that results in a less fulminant, more deteriorative clinical picture. The patient history will reveal gradual, progressive cognitive decline and loss of memory over a period of months or years. The hallmarks of dementia include a loss of adaptability, increased rigidity of response, and decreased learning and memory capacities. The fixed response patterns that emerge as a result of the disorder necessitate increased need for the patient to exercise control over the environment. Stereotypic, rigid reactions require environmental stability to prevent or offset precipitate confusion that awaits in all new situations. The ability to discard insignificant stimuli that impinge from the environment is lost.

The history will often reveal a pattern of failing self-care activities, and general decline over the past few months or years. Personality may reflect an accentuation of premorbid traits, or a narrowing and shallowness of affect. Mood may be either generally flattened or labile. Thought processes and behavior appear significantly slowed. Patients tire easily, their habits deteriorate, and shortened attention spans prevent any extended pursuit of activities. Apathetic withdrawal is common, in part to avoid any direct confrontation with overly demanding situations.

Judgment is impaired, and is often the first manifestation of dementia. Memory impairment is greater for recent than remote events. The patient may forget the examiner's name within minutes, and often forgets instructions within seconds; if asked to stand up and cross the room to open the door, the patient might pause puzzled after a few steps, having forgotten what the examiner's request was. Preoccupation with remote events can be as great as recent memory loss, and there may be frequent confusion of past and immediate circumstances.

Disorientation to time and place, and later to person, may often suggest some wish fulfillment. Asked to state where she is, the patient may indicate "at home" or "work," rather than in the hospital, and persist in the disorientation. Persistence here, like avoidance of other demanding or challenging encounters, suggests a profound need to ward off anxiety that accompanies any situation that poses failure or catastrophic threat.

Prominent Features of Chronic Organic Mental Syndrome

History

The onset is gradual and progressive over months or years. There is evidence of failing personal and social capacities. Evidence of failing cognitive and mnemonic skills is apparent.

Interview Questions

Since the state of the patient's household can be a good indicator of capacity for self-care, Sloane (1980) recommends interviewing family and friends prior to the patient, and asking certain pertinent questions:

- Does the patient live alone?
- When was the patient last competent?
- Was the onset sudden? What has been the course since?
- Is the patient mobile? How much self-care is the patient capable of?

Behavior

The patient may display impaired judgment, as well as disorientation to time and place, stereotypic, rigid reactions, and concrete inflexibility in thought. There is a marked slowness of thought, a flattened or labile affect, and nocturnal confusion and wandering. Impaired memory, bowel and bladder incontinence, and ideational impoverishment are also evident.

Clinical Stages

Constantinidis (1978) has identified four stages of concurring defects of language, praxis, and gnosis in the patient with dementia. First is the inability to find the right word (constructional graphic apraxia in the form of impaired ability to reproduce perspective). Also present is a difficulty recognizing pictures of things, and digital autotopagnosia (loss of ability to identify own body parts). Second is paraphrases, a loss of perspective in graphic praxic constructual reproduction, and difficulty copying complicated hand gestures. In the third stage patients substitute incorrect words, can no longer draw cubes in two dimensions, make mistakes of articulation in constructual graphic reproduction, show ideomotor praxic difficulty copying conventional symbolic gestures, and display bilateral stereognosic difficulty (loss of object recognition by touch). In the fourth stage they make mistakes when forming individual words, link unrelated parts of the model together in drawing, show ideomotor and ideatory apraxia, display body auto-topagnosia, and have a loss of normal reaction to pain.

Neurologic Signs

The neurologic examination provides invaluable data that, in concordance with a complete physical and mental status assessment, provides a reasonably comprehensive data base. The neurological examination should take into account the physiological changes that have accompanied normal aging: diminished vibratory sense in the lower extremities, particularly at the ankles; reduced pain and touch sensitivity; a general decrease in sensory acuity; restriction of upward gaze; loss of fine coordination; and the fact that ankle jerks are often absent. The exam should include evaluation of overall level of consciousness, and testing for primitive reflexes and sensory perception that will reflect diffuse cerebral dysfunction. Habot and Libow (1980) recommend that the examiner include the possibility of decreased hearing and vision, slow motor responses, weakness, decreased memory, fear of failure, and language barrier as factors that may bias the assessment process.

Gait is often impaired in the elderly and may be particularly revealing of any neurologic deterioration.

Primitive reflexes such as the palmomental, or snouting, sucking, and grasping, are physiological, and are universally present in the human infant at birth. They disappear with CNS maturation and the development of inhibitory mechanisms in the adult, but reappear in old age, dementia, and certain neurologic disorders. Abnormal reflex responses include grasping, sucking, snouting, and the palmomental, nuchocephalic, corneomandibular, and glabella tap reflexes. Although the result of the neurologic exam may be normal for many demented patients, particularly during the early stages of the disease, neurologic signs that have been shown to correlate with the presence of diffuse cerebral dysfunction and should be tested include:

- Paratonic rigidity—generalized resistance to passive movement by a counterpull, present throughout the entire range of movement. Usually a manifestation of bilateral cortical disease.
- Motor impersistence—inability to sustain positions such as keeping the eyes closed for 15 seconds.
- Corneomandibular reflex—deflection of the lower jaw to one side when, with the subject's mouth open, the cornea of the opposite eye is irritated.
- Glabella blink—light tapping on the glabellar region from above produces a positive, nonfatiguing blinking.
- Nuchocephalic reflex—while briskly turning the shoulders to the right or left while standing, the head retains its original position instead of turning normally in the direction of the shoulders.
- Snouting—sharp, brief pressure to the closed lips, produces a positive puckering movement.

- Grasping—stroking the palm, especially the region between the thumb and index finger, produces a positive grasping or closing of the hand.
- Sucking—stroking the oral region or placing an object between the lips produces a positive puckering or sucking motion.
- Palmomental reflex—stroking the thenar eminence of the hand produces a positive contraction of the chin's ipsilateral mentalis muscle, and wrinkling of the skin.

According to Wang (1981) neurological signs such as these include the presence of pathological (or the reappearance of certain primitive reflex responses), and the presence of deficits in sensory or motor function, depending upon where the brain tissue is most affected. Several reflexes (grasping, sucking) are the "frontal release" reflexes, considered characteristic of frontal lobe dysfunction. Others, such as glabellar blink, are related more to diffuse brain dysfunction or subcortical lesions.

Neuropsychologic Features

Language

In approximately 90 percent of any patient population, damage to the left hemisphere results in aphasia. Related disorders may involve motor aspects of language, such as dysarthria (disarticulation), dysphasia, or paraphasia (using the wrong word). Dysphasias may be fluent, in which case the patient has good articulation but frequent paraphasias, or nonfluent, in which case poor articulation, sparse output, but nonetheless meaningful content, is produced only with difficulty. Impairments like these may be identified by asking the patient to describe commonplace objects (e.g., a watch, ring, cup, or hand). The patient may be able to describe the usage of the item, but unable to name it correctly. Asking the patient to write, read aloud, and repeat words, phrases, or digits, or comprehend simple sequential instructions (pick up the spoon, walk to the door), provides simple and easily assessed estimations of language function.

Attention

Variability of attention should be assessed to differentiate the brain damaged patient from patients whose attention is distracted because of task, ideosyncractic, or functional causes. According to Mattis (1976) lateral inattention or lateral spatial neglect is seen in patients with parietal lobe lesions contralateral to the neglected side. This type of inattention is not seen in patients with a structurally intact CNS. Affected patients behave, especially following a stroke, as if they neither receive nor process information that alerts them to deficits. The presence of lateral spatial neglect can be considered both a sensitive and localizing sign of brain damage.

Conceptualization

Concretized thought is a sensitive yet less localizing sign of brain damage. When asked to name three things to eat, the patient may say soup, tea, and carrots. When then asked how the soup, tea, and carrots are alike, the patient may respond, "They're not alike." The failure to identify the three items as food indicates concreteness of thought. What is also demonstrated is the fact that while deductive reasoning remains intact, the inability to categorize items suggests that inductive capacities are diminished (Mattis, 1976).

Visual–Spatial Perception

Patients with posterior lesions show distortions in size determination, in orientation of the target stimulus, and in figure–ground relations. Mattis suggests that visual "noise" (e.g., a line drawn across the face of a clock) will reduce the patient's ability to identify the stimulus properly. In severe spatial distortion, even the absence of visual noise will not prevent incorrect responses. Patients with posterior lesions, particularly of the right hemisphere (nondominant), have significant difficulty processing visual information. To assess the person's visual–spatial and constructional ability ask him to draw simple figures, forms, or parts of a whole, and the relationship of the parts to one another and the whole (e.g., children at a picnic, friends in an exercise class).

Face–Hand Test

The patient's face and hand are stimulated, first ipsilaterally and then contralaterally. The patient is then asked to state where the touch occurs, or whether the touch occurs in one or two places. A variety of ipsilateral and contralateral trials using the patient and the examiner are repeated, with the patient asked to localize the stimuli. The test is quite sensitive, and in the absence of any errors cerebral damage is unlikely. Parietal lobe lesions, however, may result in raised sensation thresholds or distortion of somatosensory data processing. Errors reported by Verwoerdt (1981) include:

- failing to report touch to the hand (extinction)
- localizing hand touch to the knee or elsewhere (displacement)
- pointing to the examiner's hand (projection)
- pointing into space (exsomesthesia)

Extinction of facial touch is rare and suggestive of a functional disorder.

Memory

Assessment of immediate and short-term memory may be undertaken fairly simply by asking the patient to repeat a series of 5 or 7 digits, or simple sentences such as "The black horse galloped" or "The silver airplane landed smoothly." The patient must be attentive, so that when asked within a few minutes to repeat the sentence it can be recalled. Mattis (1976) indicates that frontal lesions and diffuse cortical lesions will not generally result in impairment of remote memory. However, in the presence of concretized thought and perseveration (the hallmarks of frontal lobe syndrome), impairment of encoding processes for precise storage and inflexible retrieval strategies is evident, and creates mnemonic behavior commonly seen in dementia patients.

Dyspraxia

Dyspraxia should be assessed by asking the patient to carry out simple but purposeful movements such as snapping the fingers or crossing the legs. In the presence of an ideomotor apraxia the patient who is well able to feed himself and ambulate adequately may be unable to pretend to eat soup, open a door.

Intellect

Any truly comprehensive assessment of the patient must include accurate estimations of intelligence. The fact that this is frequently not undertaken is compounded by other measurement problems as well. The Wechsler Adult Intelligence Scale (WAIS) deterioration index, which compares *hold* (tending to remain stable) scales with *don't hold* (declining with age) scales is quite simply computed; the sum of the *don't hold* scales is subtracted from the sum of the *holds,* and then divided by the sum of *holds.* In addition to the deterioration index, the degree of dispersion of scores, or scatter, between and within each subscale indicates either decline (as with age), or psychopathology. A high degree of scatter has been reported for functionally psychotic patients, and has been well documented for brain damaged patients. In addition, performance IQ is known to decline more than verbal IQ with age. Studies that compared normal elderly with organic brain syndrome patients revealed differences in patterned responses, but Schaie and Schaie (1977) and Miller (1981) report that no conclusive intellectual differences were found. The underlying assumption by poorly informed health professionals that the psychological consequences of dementia or brain damage are similar to those of normal aging has not, to date, been supported in the literature.

Comparisons of normal aging and clinical syndromes (either functional or organic) have been hampered by the generalized lack of reliable norms for older groups. Attempts at subjective estimations of premorbid IQ in dementia have been equally unsatisfactory. Given the lack of normative data for normal aging, and the present inability to determine whether declines can be attributed to age-related deficits or organic pathology, assessment through the use of reading tests that tap less fragile verbal skills is recommended. It is equally recommendable that clinicians avoid all assumptions of intellectual impairment until substantive, objective data can be obtained. Most longitudinal studies have suggested that the pattern of intellectual decline in old age has been exaggerated (Miller, 1981; Schaie & Schaie, 1977).

Certain tools have been determined to be especially valuable in assessment of mental functions in organic mental syndrome. The Short Portable Mental Status questionnaire (SPMSQ) and Face–Hand test, both of which are brief and easily administered, have been reported to be the most useful. Accurate assessment depends more on determining the presence or absence of significant cognitive deficits than on any other factor, and health care providers are encouraged to obtain professional psychometric assistance, and to seek guidance in developing and using clinically meaningful tools as the need arises. They are also encouraged to continue to assess the elderly patient as long as possible, well beyond what Small (1973) calls the "immutability of neurological disorders"—the pessimistic notion that all such disorders doom the patient to an unchangeable lifelong limitation. The compensatory mechanisms employed by "demented" patients are often varied and challenging for the clinician.

Key Concepts Regarding Chronic Organic Mental Syndrome

The following is a list of important concepts to be kept in mind during the assessment process.

- A gradual, insidious onset
- A progressive deterioration of personal, social, or occupational functions
- A general decline in intellectual function
- A decreased flexibility in thought
- An increased rigidity in thought and behavior
- A marked slowness of thought and behavior
- Impaired memory
- Impaired judgment
- Disturbed higher cortical functions (aphasia, apraxia, agnosia)
- An alteration or accentuation of premorbid personality
- Nocturnal confusion and wandering
- Bowel and bladder incontinence
- Disorientation to time, place, and later to person
- Compulsive orderliness

SUMMARY

Acute organic mental syndrome in the aged often presents with fulminating fluctuations in mentation and behavior. If detected early this reversible condition, which may result from underlying systemic disease, drugs, trauma, surgery, etc., usually offers a favorable response to treatment. If untreated, however, it may progress to irreversible, chronic organic mental syndrome.

Chronic organic syndrome is characterized by its insidious onset and progressive deterioration of cognitive and behavioral functions. Steady decline in general self-care activities, and a slowing of thought processes and behavior, are characteristic. The clinical stages of the disorder's progress, and the importance of the neurological examination as part of the overall assessment of physical and mental status, are discussed.

Neuropsychologic features of the assessment process include appraisal of language ability, attention variability, conceptualization, visual–spatial perception, somatosensory processes (through the face–hand test), memory, and dyspraxia. Brief, simple, and clinically applicable examples have been suggested. Psychometric study of intellectual decline and chronic organic mental syndrome continues, but the need for substantive, differentiating data, and normative data on the intellectual abilities of the healthy aged person, remains a pressing concern of those involved in assessment of the aged patient.

REFERENCES

Constantinidis, J. (1978). Is Alzheimer's disease a major form of senile dementia? Clinical, anatomical, and genetic data. In R. Katzman, R. Terry, & K. Bick (Eds.), *Alzheimer's disease: Senile dementia and related disorders. Aging series, vol. 7* (pp. 15–25). New York: Raven Press.

Habot, B. & Libow, L., (1980). The interrelationship of mental and physical status and its assessment in the older adult: Mind-Body interaction. In J. Birren & R. Sloane (Eds.), *Handbook of mental health and aging* (pp. 701–716). Englewood Cliffs, NJ: Prentice-Hall, Inc.

Mattis, S. (1976). Mental status examination for organic mental syndrome in the elderly patient. In L. Bellak & T. Karasu (Eds.), *Geriatric psychiatry* (pp. 77–101). New York: Grune and Stratton.

Miller, E. (1981). The differential psychological evaluation. In N. Miller & G. Cohen (Eds.), *Clinical aspects of Alzheimer's disease and senile dementia. Aging series, vol. 15* (pp. 121–138). New York: Raven Press.

Schaie, K. & Schaie, J. (1977). Clinical assessment and aging. In J. Birren & K. Schaie (Eds.), *Handbook of the psychology of aging* (pp. 692–723). New York: Van Nostrand Reinhold Company.

Sloane, R. (1980). Organic brain syndrome. In J. Birren & R. Sloane (Eds.), *Handbook of mental health and aging* (pp. 554–590). Englewood Cliffs, NJ: Prentice-Hall, Inc.

Small, L. (1973). *Neuropsychodiagnosis in psychotherapy*. New York: Brunner/Mazel.

Verwoerdt, A. (1976). *Clinical geropsychiatry*. Baltimore: Williams and Wilkins Co.

Wang, H. (1981). Neuropsychiatric procedures for the assessment of Alzheimer's disease, senile dementia, and related disorders. In N. Miller & G. Cohen (Eds.), *Clinical aspects of Alzheimer's disease and senile dementia. Aging series, vol. 15* (pp. 85–101). New York: Raven Press.

SUGGESTED READINGS

Feinberg, I. (1975). Chronic brain syndrome. In I. Glick (Ed.), *Syllabus—introduction to clinical psychiatry* (pp. 46–54). San Francisco: University of California.

Podlone, M. & Millikan, C. (1981). Neurology. In M. O'Hara-Devereaux, L. Andrus, & C. Scott (Eds.), *Edlercare—a guide to clinical geriatrics* (pp. 115–134). New York: Grune & Stratton, Inc.

PART III

Guidelines for Intervention

The resolution of fundamental social problems, such as poverty, aging, or crime, can require inordinate amounts of time and effort. This is partly due to the manner in which problem resolution is approached. Although rapid change is a byword of modern life, problem solving strategies often lack any farsighted plan designed with the present problem and its future consequences in mind.

More often than not these fundamental social problems are separated as entities unto themselves, rather like diagnostic categories. They are seen as essentially quite disparate problems requiring different solutions. Watzlawick, Weakland, and Fisch (1974) point out that often the next step is to create enormous administrative structures and industries of expertise, which produces instead vast numbers of incompetent individuals. They contend that this basically counterproductive approach is too often used.

Change can be implemented effectively by focusing on minimal, concrete goals, going slowly, and proceeding step by step, rather than strongly promoting vast and vague targets with whose desirability nobody would take issue, but whose attainability is a different question altogether.

With an eye toward present problems and adumbrations of the future, Part III examines selected guidelines for psychotherapeutic, chemotherapeutic, and sociotherapeutic intervention in mental health and aging.

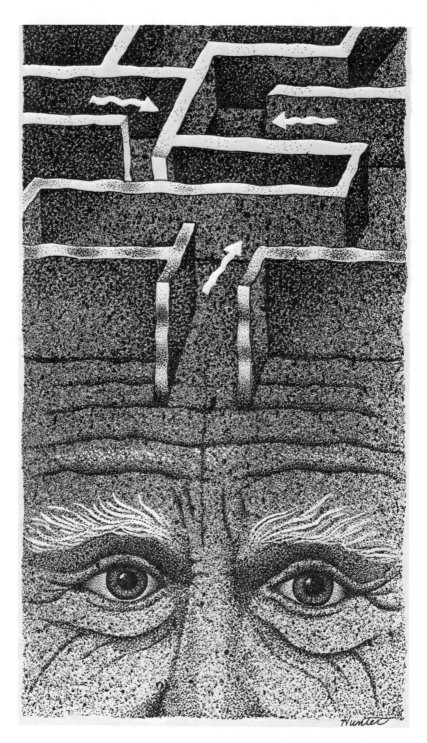

Chapter 9

Psychotherapy

Individual, group, family, milieu, and social learning approaches to the mental health problems of later life all offer different yet equally effective guidelines for psychotherapeutic intervention. The selection of one approach over another is determined by the specific treatment needs of patients, the prevailing psychotherapeutic philosophy of the nurse, and the nature of mental disorders presented.

The older adult brings to the treatment scene diminished awareness of stress as an etiological agent, sensory deficits that shape and alter patient–nurse communication, and little familiarity with the psychodynamic process. Focal interventions must address the patient's conflict with anomie, identity loss, mortality, and senescence. Many approaches, have been found to be decidedly beneficial, and this chapter examines several of proven effectiveness.

DYADIC APPROACHES

The stereotypic pessimism attached to the supposed inability of older clients to benefit from psychotherapy has by now been largely dispelled. Most elderly persons are receptive to psychotherapy and cannot in all fairness be described as categorically inflexible. They are motivated to resolve problems, redirect energies into constructive outlets, and attempt to find meaning in life.

Knight's (1978) review of research on the efficacy of various schools of psychotherapeutic thought shows that successful resolution is possible from diverse approaches. Traditional and modified forms of psychoanalysis, Jungian analysis, gestalt therapy, as well as eclectic approaches, have all proven effective. Combinations of biological (drug or nutritional therapy) and psychosocial (milieu therapy) approaches are also beneficial.

The negative attitude that originally pervaded geriatric psychotherapy can be traced to two principal sources; the elderly who were traditionally reluctant to seek mental health services, and delayed entering the mental health system until symptoms achieved crises proportions, and the cost of psychotherapy, which placed it well beyond the reach of the average older adult. Because a significant percentage still fall below the poverty level, income imposes a major barrier to those elderly patients in need of help. Due to differences in reporting strategy, estimates vary, but recent figures reveal that only 2–4 percent of all persons seen in outpatient clinics are over 65. Knight also reports that several studies indicate that those receiving care may not be the ones who need it most.

The goals of psychotherapy for the older adult include reducing the fear of obsolescence and death, undoing the noxious influences of public attitude and policy, reducing stress-related anxiety, short-term relief of specific medical disorders, acceptance of the aging process, promotion of personal growth, reality counseling to decrease disorientation, and the development of friendships to facilitate adjustment.

Of particular importance in the selection of therapeutic goals is the recent expansion of the nurse's treatment philosophy, from what was once a preclusive emphasis on documented pathology to a balanced identification of assets and liabilities. The latter view enables the patient and nurse to identify and summon those resources still available for use. Cognizance of the interactive effect of mind and body, of increased meaningless and devaluation of life, and of sensory and communication loss, is central to any balanced estimation.

Communication Therapy

Virtually all psychosocial activities are mediated by verbal behavior and, consequently, communication becomes the single most vital element in all dyadic and nondyadic intervention. The importance of communication as a vehicle for the fulfillment of life and for the establishment of interpersonal relationships in later life cannot be overemphasized. Bloomer (1960) stresses the significance of verbal communication in all aspects of life; acceptance within groups, emotional release, memory, conveyance of information, and philosophical interpretation. At its most basic, psychotherapy *is* therapeutic communication; because of the aged patient's sensory, intellectual, and central nervous system deficits, the identification of therapeutic goals must begin with assessment of communicative skill.

Many elderly clients have communication difficulties. Comprehension and response to questions require more time. Treatment instructions may be forgotten. The nurse must speak slowly and clearly (not necessarily loudly), exchanges may have to be repeated, and instructions written down. Verbal language and metacommunication (nonverbal, paralingual, and body language) assume greater significance with this patient population. Awareness of facial expressions and the emotional tone of word patterns can hasten interaction beyond protective superficiality toward early problem identification.

Despite difficulties, every effort should be made to establish and maintain dialogue directly with the patient rather than accompanying family members. The temptation to bypass or disregard the patient's message in preference to easier dialogues must be avoided, since even inadvertently it may undermine the progress of treatment. The goals of communication therapy include appraisal of present communicative skills level, application of verbal and metacommunication strategies to establish clear channels of message transmission, and the development of an interpersonal alliance in which meaningful, motivating, and self-reinforcing communication can occur. Either individual or group formats can be used to achieve these goals.

Insight Therapy

Insight-oriented approaches frequently use the therapist in an active role to encourage the expression of feelings and interpretations, a process Verwoerdt (1976) describes as an in-depth learning experience for both patient and therapist. The goal of this therapy is less clearly outlined, so effective functioning in the patient is expected to result from a more time-consuming personality reconstruction. Intrapsychic alterations enable the ego to emerge as a more mature and effective mental agency. Maladaptive defenses and character rigidity become consciously recognized. Early memories are reactivated and explored. Feelings that have been mobilized in association with memory may result in the identification of elements of personality that are either constructive or destructive for the individual.

Supportive Therapy

Supportive approaches include the encouragement of maximal use of the patient's psychological assets through strengthened defenses, improved control mechanisms, and restored equilibrium, resulting in the replacement of maladaptive defenses with more adaptive ones. Confidence and trust in the nurse are essential to the success of supportive therapy. Practical interpersonal and situationally defined problems are examined, with attention to realistic solutions that will incorporate the patient's present abilities and constraints. The clarification of problems can often take place without the elimination of underlying guilt, anger, or fear. The nurse's role includes emphasis on teaching, and the learner is encouraged to arrive at a personal solution.

The question of independence versus dependence is sometimes raised within the context of supportive therapy. The patient must be allowed to utilize regression if and when it makes possible the acceptance of dependency as a means of accepting help from others, in addition to instilling the hope, security, and reassurance so essential to well being. The unearthing of certain dependence needs in the course of treatment may permit some persons to cope more effectively, and should not be categorically dismissed.

NONDYADIC APPROACHES

Group Work

A basic rule of group work with the elderly, and one that promotes reorientation and sensory awareness, requires that every person recognize the other members at every meeting by greeting and touching. The benefits in terms of feeling recognized by name and making physical contact add much to the sense of mutual collaboration in the goals of the group.

The group leader must be able to face his or her own feelings about loss, physical and social limitations, incapacitating illness, and death. Failure of the leader to face these issues will make it virtually impossible for other patients to come to grips with them.

Younger nurses working with older patients must work through their own counter-transference feelings toward parents and grandparents who are contemporaries of the group. Two approaches that have been found most beneficial in this regard are regularly scheduled experiential groups for staff members (in which they examine unresolved conflicts over aging and death, guilt feelings about their youth, and the significance of group experience), and regularly scheduled staff participation in aged groups to increase awareness of each other as members.

Berger and Berger (1972) cite the eligibility requirements for member participation in outpatient group therapy:

1. The patient has the ability to walk, be wheeled, or escorted to the center.
2. The patient is functioning in the "here and now".
3. The patient is not unmanageable, or prevented by undirected restlessness from sitting still.
4. The patient does not suffer from unremitting bowel and bladder incontinence or advanced deafness.
5. The patient is willing to participate voluntarily.
6. The patient is able to recognize and acknowledge the need for emotional or psychological help.
7. The patient is able to understand the language used in the group.

The locus in which group therapy is conducted often determines the goals and aims of that therapy. Within the institution, the focus may be on preparing for discharge, reducing patient management problems, ameliorating disruptive behavior, improving morale, assessing or restructuring attitudes, improving adaptation to the institutional environment, improving interpersonal relationships, or reducing personal suffering.

Within the locus of the community, a more flexible and adaptable membership is seen, with emphasis on personal growth and life enrichment. The application of group principles to preretirement and retirement problems and improved personal, familial, or social function is very common. Comprehensive community mental health programs also provide a wide network of agency-extended group opportunities. Neighborhood community centers, churches, homes for the aged, civic recreation departments, and ancillary community institutions offer a whole host of group approaches to therapy for the aged.

The extent to which certain topics are discussed in the group and the depth given to that discussion is determined, according to Ross (1975) by a classification system of group modalities that are linked to patient needs, with interaction occurring at increasing depth levels. Guideposts for discussion include the specific aims of the practitioner for each member and group, the depth level desired, and group techniques used by the leader. Five major group foci include:

- activity–catharsis–mastery—work groups that foster opportunities for reaching out, touching, exploration of materials, and occupational therapy resulting in catharsis, tension channeling, and ego mastery
- cognitive–information—groups emphasizing educational models, family life models, and occupational or recreational skills
- interpersonal–socialization—groups that focus on security, belonging, and companionship
- relationship–experiential—diagnostic and treatment groups working through social rehabilitation clinics, halfway house programs, and in medical or psychiatric settings
- uncovering–introspective—psychotherapeutic groups with an emphasis on improved functioning via personality reconstruction

Sensory Stimulation

Because of the alterations and deficits within the neurosensory system, a balance between sensory stimulation and deprivation is desired. Most often conducted in group settings, sensory stimulation attempts to provide optimal arousal of visual, auditory, taste, smell, tactile, and thermal apparatuses. Sound (music, birdsong), touch (fabric texture, sand), smell (perfume, flowers), taste (jello, pickles, potato chips), sight (candlelight, near and distant objects, colored pictures), and thermal (ice, heating pad) sensitivity are all explored in an effort to reawaken sensory acuity. The simplest techniques, even as mundane as sharing candy among group members, can be effective in stimulating sensory awareness. Socialization skills are improved, and a heightened awareness of sensory acuity increases a sense of personal functional autonomy.

Activity Therapy

Activity therapy attempts to stimulate and focus attention around a particular form of interaction. The techniques employed are intended to create a vivid and stimulating environment which motivation, independent expression, and self-assertiveness will be manifest. Drama, dance and movement, music, poetry reading and writing, physical exercise and sports, creative writing, autobiographical and oral history, are among the several approaches commonly used. Activity therapy differs from recreational activity in its therapeutic focus on verbal and nonverbal expression of *problems* that are described and responded to as part of the activity. Hartford (1980) reports the psychological benefits of body movement and dance therapy. Deliberately created and introduced interpretive dance steps were found to aid elderly women in emotional expression. Music has been found to serve as a psychic energizer which, when combined with rhythmics, activates regressed and even brain-damaged elderly patients, thereby assisting in the development of a stronger sense of social awareness.

Physical activity is crucial to the older adult. Motor inactivity in the osteoporotic-prone patient hastens decalification, while activity strengthens motor integrity; regular exercise programs enable the patient to gain greater control over the body movements than would be otherwise possible. The psychological gain from improved mobility is seen in stronger independent self-care activities and personal instrumentality.

Reality Orientation

Reality orientation efforts are directed specifically to the needs of confused and memory-disorded chronic brain syndrome patients. Continual reiteration of basic personal and current information is used to reorientate patients. Those who demonstrate transitory periods of confusion, with intermittent periods of clarity, are best helped by these techniques. Groups of six or fewer members respond better, since individualized attention is often necessary. The patient's name, location, age, the current date, names of staff members, other patients, and relatives, are all repeated frequently. Continuity is important, so material that was covered in previous sessions is repeated. Patients are rewarded for every success. As clarity increases, subsequent sessions address current events, history, and geographical information relevant to the patient. All staff with whom the patient is in contact are involved in the therapy and are instructed to continue it during normal daily activities. The patient is reminded of immediate experience in descriptive words that help reorientation to simple aspects of the environment.

Resocialization–Remotivation

Resocialization–remotivation groups can be particularly effective for older adults with varying degrees of cerebral impairment. The emotional disorganization accompanying brain damage often leads to the misconception that group treatment is futile, but such groups have repeatedly been found to help patients orient themselves better to their environment.

The aim of remotivation is improvement of patients who are withdrawn and apathetic by means of relating to and communicating with others. The group goal is normal healthy behavior and verbalization. The success of remotivation in the reestablishment of identity, reduction of depression, and even significant improvement in staff morale and attitudes following remotivation techniques with patients, have all been well documented (Butler, 1970; Hartford, 1980).

Similar to remotivation, the aim of resocialization is the relearning of basic social skills and instrumentalities necessary to daily life. Short-term applications of resocialization techniques have been quite successful, not only in improving instrumental skills, but in enabling members to identify and vent feelings. A climate of mutual trust and freedom from retaliation is essential, allowing members to use catharsis to ease tension, release negative emotions, develop supportive relationships, and develop environmentally appropriate behavior.

Reminiscence and Life Review

The life review involves a detailed life history that, when explored, aids in the attainment of understanding and appreciation of the sense of continuity of life that is essential in the face of myriad changes associated with old age. The process provides a sense of meaning in life. Reminiscence and review involve the integration of one's actual life with the way in which it might have been lived. Reminiscences recall the facts of an individual life, and weaves them into a harmonious perspective to achieve a sense of closure; writing a ''revised'' autobiography to be left behind for those who come after. Butler (1970) believes that when the life review proceeds in an adaptive manner and the patient's ego surveys and reflects on the past

> new meanings are assigned to past experiences based on a new, larger perspective of life; the individual is able to come to terms with regret; guilt and loss may be worked through; understanding of life is expanded; understanding of self within life experience is enhanced; preparation for death with less fear is greater.

The life review process is not without hazards, since mild regret may become more severe and lead to despair, anxiety, or guilt. Obsessive ruminations, panic, and even suicidal preoccupation are threats to be guarded against, particularly with the isolated elderly who may sense life's losses more acutely and believe their lives are wasted. Successful completion of the process, however, can result in constructive personality reorganization, creativity, wisdom, atonement, contentment, maturity, and autonomy.

Gestalt–Fantasy–Psychodrama

Veridical or experiential learning opportunities provided by gestalt, fantasy, or psychodrama techniques, have been proven valuable in expanding the older individual's sense of creative imagination. They allow the patient to move beyond senses and body experience to discover new dimensions of the self. Adult free play in fantasy permits a vicarious journey into events otherwise impossible. Gestalt techniques provide a sharpening of thoughts, emotions, and perceptions of the self in new, nontraditional ways, frequently overcoming insipient feelings of powerlessness.

Psychodramatic methods, such as *doubling* or *the magic shop,* permit the aged group member to reenact events to explore alternative endings. Exercises such as the *unconscious mind mirror,* in which the patient establishes and alters an imaginery mirror image, can be useful in restoring a more positive physical image. Like videotape feedback methods, which are also used, the reaffirmation of positive body image is greatly enhanced by techniques that give freedom of direction to the individual and expand self awareness.

Family Therapy

The role of aged family member holds varied meanings, defined according to family circumstances. Smith, Lelong, and Adelberg (1981) have found that the younger family members find the old, frail parent to be a new responsibility (at a time in life when their own needs are increasing). They look into a mirror of their own aging and mortality; this may cause unrealistic guilt at having neglected parents or having failed to prevent their aging, or it may bring forth love for parents who once constituted an entire universe in the child's mind's eye. It may mean sadness at those who were once powerful losing all power, and it often means hostility at parents who dare to need and demand so much.

Verwoerdt (1976) adds an additional note. "The stresses of chronic illness and hospitalization frequently have the unfortunate result of depleting the family's economic resources as well as its reservoir of good will." The emotional velocity of the combination of aged parent with chronic illness often evokes somewhat primal responses.

Slater (1969) believes that the attitudes of parent and child toward hospitalization are surprisingly reminiscent of people in more primitive cultures to sorcery. An almost magical fear of "catching old age" can be observed beneath the family's intense need to insulate the aged member in a hospital. The sense of benevolent protection is often totally inappropriate to the realities of the situation.

Filial maturity, as Spark and Brody (1972) use the term, refers to the mature adult's capacity to be depended on by the patient, thereby marking a healthy transition from genital maturity to old age. Instead of a simple role reversal, the process requires fulfillment of the filial role rather than adopting a "parental" role with one's own parent, and implies resolution of earlier transitional phases of life. It requires the adult child to resolve conflicts about what cannot be done to aid the aged parent, in addition to mature acceptance of that which can and should be done in the filial role. To relieve guilt on the one hand and help the adult child behave responsibly on the other is the family therapist's difficult task.

Milieu Therapy

Milieu therapy involves the entire staff and patient population in a therapeutic coalition. Young and old patients are integrated in programs that attempt to instill mutual stimulation and interaction. The benefits of integration tend to offset the regressive features of fixation in an extended role of illness so common to the aged. The therapeutic community provides meaningful tasks and makes reasonable demands, all designed to enable the patient to work purposively, relate to others, and make independent decisions. In addition, individuality and dignity are reinforced by the patient's use of personal belongings and clothes, and direct collaboration in all community decision making.

Social Learning Approaches

Social learning methods are increasingly viewed as effective tools for the extinction of dysfunctional or disruptive behavior and the reinforcement of appropriate behavior. Maladaptive behaviors are considered to be learned response habits that have become part of character. The modification or reversal of behavior utilizes learning techniques such as extinction, desensitization, operant conditioning, negative reinforcement, and counterconditioning. Improvement in social functioning through the use of social learning approaches has been reported by Berni and Fordyce (1977) and Schonfield (1980). The former authors cite the case of one elderly woman with Parkinsonism who frequently lost her balance in her wheelchair and fell so far to the left that she was unable to regain her balance. A restraint belt was all that prevented her from falling to the floor. Operant conditioning and the installation of an electric eye on the back of her wheelchair produced dramatic improvement. When her head and shoulders moved a very few inches to the left in the earliest stages of a fall, a tone was sounded. After she had heard the tone a few times she was able to realign herself and prevent the fall. During an observation period of 12 days she went from a rate of 20 falls per hour to none.

Schonfield cites the case of two male nursing home patients aged 92 and 85 who were persuaded to forego use of their wheelchairs as transportation to the dining room simply by asking them to do so, and then rewarding them with praise and a chat en route. When the patients were told not to walk, and reinforcement was withdrawn, they reverted to the wheelchairs.

SUMMARY

Older adults are now known to benefit from various forms of psychotherapy. Because of predisposing sensory, psychological, and social function losses, attention to communication processes is essential. Dyadic and nondyadic approaches enable the older adult to identify dysfunctional behaviors, expand the existing repertoir of coping strategies, and learn how to resolve the dilemmas of late life.

Group approaches are particularly beneficial, not only in economic terms, but in enabling the individual to discover that problems are, indeed, universally shared. Sensory stimulation techniques and activity therapy provide a strong contextual base for the exploration of problems.

Reminiscence and life review provide opportunities for reappraisal of one's life, thereby gaining a richer sense of meaning, resolution, and mutuality. Family therapy enables members to reexamine traditional roles, seek resolutions to feelings of responsibility for the aged family member's condition, and resolve underlying conflicts regarding filial maturity and institutionalization.

Milieu therapy includes the aged patient in therapeutic community activities that attempt to prevent extended sick role and dependent behavior. Social learning approaches have been remarkably effective in targeting and treating specific dysfunctional behaviors, and offer considerable promise in future work with aged patients.

REFERENCES

Berger, M. & Berger, L. (1972). Psychogeriatric group approaches. In C. Sager & H. Kaplan (Eds.), *Progress in group and family therapy* (pp. 726–736). New York: Brunner/Mazel

Berni, R. & Fordyce, W. (1977). *Behavior modification and the nursing process.* St. Louis: C. V. Mosby.

Bloomer, H. (1960). Communication problems among aged county hospital patients. *Geriatrics, 15,* 291–295.

Butler, R. (1970). Looking forward to what? The life review, legacy and excessive identity versus change. *American Behavioral Sciences, 14,* 121–128.

Hartford, M. (1980). The use of group methods for work with the aged. In J. Birren & R. Sloane (Eds.), *Handbook of mental health and aging* (pp. 806–826). Englewood Cliffs, NJ: Prentice-Hall, Inc.

Knight, B. (1978). Psychotherapy and behavior change with the non-institutionalized aged. *International Journal of Aging and Human Development, 9*(3), 221–236.

Ross, M. (1975). Community geriatric group therapies: A comprehensive review. In M. Rosenbaum & M. Berger (Eds.), *Group psychotherapy and group function* (pp. 500–520). New York: Basic Books, Inc.

Schonfield, A. (1980). Learning, memory, and aging. In J. Birren & R. Sloane (Eds.), *Handbook of mental health and aging* (pp. 214–244). Englewood Cliffs, NJ: Prentice-Hall, Inc.

Slater, P. (1969). Cross-cultural views of the aged. In R. Kastenbaum (Ed.), *New thoughts on old age* (pp. 229–236). New York: Springer Publishing Company.

Smith, B., Lelong, J., & Adelberg, B. (1981). *Aging parents and dilemmas of their children.* Austin, Texas: Hogg Foundation for Mental Health, The University of Texas.

Spark, G. & Brody, E. (1972). The aged are family members. In C. Sager & H. Kaplan (Eds.), *Progress in group and family therapy* (pp. 712–725). New York: Brunner/Mazel.

Verwoerdt, A. (1976). *Clinical geropsychiatry* (p. 140). Baltimore: Williams and Wilkins Co.

Watzlawick, P., Weakland, J. & Fisch, R. (1974). *Change: Principles of problem formation and problem resolution.* New York: W.W. Norton Company.

SUGGESTED READINGS

Dye, C. (1976). Counseling the older rehabilitation patient. International congress series, 393. *Proceedings of the First International Congress of Patient Counseling.* Amsterdam, The Netherlands: Exerpta Medica Foundation.

Eisdorfer, C. & Stotsky, B. (1977). Intervention, treatment and rehabilitation of psychiatric disorders. In J. Birren & K. Schaie (Eds.), *Handbook of the psychology of aging* (pp. 724–748). New York: Van Nostrand Reinhold.

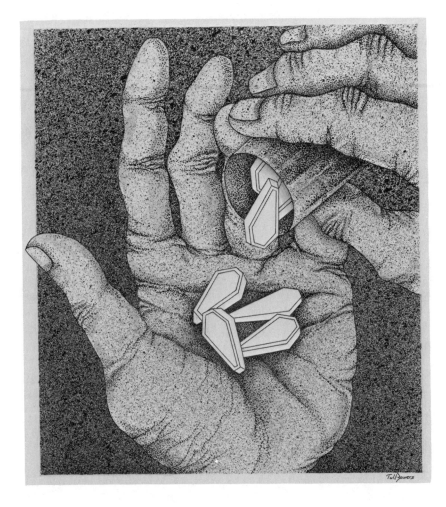

Chapter 10

Drug Therapy

Victor A. Yanchick, Ph.D.

There is a growing medical and social concern in the health care fields regarding the rational and appropriate use of drugs for the elderly. Although an estimated 11 percent of the total population in the United States is over the age of 65, Vestal (1978) and Kovar (1977) have reported that they consume nearly 30 percent of all medications, occupy over a third of all hospital beds, and account for over 29 cents of each health care dollar spent. Lamy (1980) has estimated that on the average they are given 13 prescriptions per year, mostly by internists and family practice physicians. Studies reported by Hurwitz (1969) and Williamson and Chapin (1980) indicate that they are hospitalized for adverse drug reactions twice as often as those under the age of 60. Over half of these individuals obtain their medications from repeat prescriptions that commonly involve a disproportionate amount of psychotropic agents, and ultimately are responsible for a substantial number of these adverse drug reactions. A recent study conducted in Great Britain by Kierman and Isaacs (1981) revealed that a noninstitutionalized individual over the age of 65 takes between four and five different drugs on a daily basis. The most common drug categories noted in this study were the psychotropics, the analgesic/antipyretics, and the diuretics. Less than 60 percent of the study group were considered to have accurate knowledge of the purpose of their prescriptions, and altered compliance increased significantly as the number of drugs prescribed increased. Most patients did not visit the physician who prescribed their medication when they received their last prescription, and all individuals who were taking nonprescription drugs with prescription medication admitted that they did not inform their physician that they were also consuming these products. This study points to the potential hazards that many of our older citizens encounter when they are placed on drug therapy. This situation becomes even more critical for those over the age of 80 since, according to Hurwitz (1969), the potential for

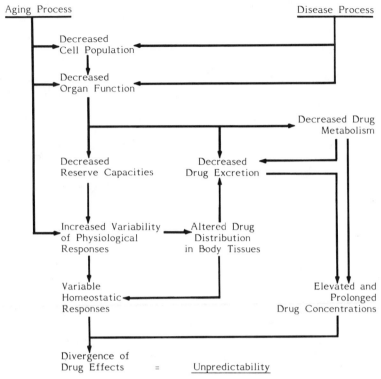

Figure 10-1. Flow diagram leading to the unpredictability of drug responses in the elderly. Adapted from Riley, 1977.

adverse drug reactions is tripled compared to individuals below the age of 50.

The high incidence of adverse drug reactions in the elderly has two distinct components, each with its own remedy. One component results from the pattern of prescribing for the elderly, and might yield to a reevaluation of prescribing habits in which symptoms are all too readily treated with drugs before the etiology is known. The other component reflects the increased propensity of older patients to react adversely to most drugs, and can be countered by more informed drug use and a greater appreciation and understanding of the many factors that can alter drug activity. In the first instance, time and the education of the health practitioner and consumer are of primary importance. The second issue is also multifaceted, and involves such factors as disease states, genetics, concomitant drug use, nutritional status, sex, biological and biochemical changes, stress, and the environment. Figure 10-1 provides a diagrammatic approach to the sequence of events that may be involved in causing unpredictable drug effects in the elderly. Although aging itself cannot be blamed as the sole biological factor explaining the association between increased drug toxicity and age, the aging process can initiate many physiological changes which increase susceptibility to disease and disability, and alter the presentation of medical conditions that may necessitate increased drug use, resulting in an increased incidence of adverse drug reactions and drug interactions. These changes may partially explain why older people appear to be more sensitive to many drugs, although the reasons for these observed age-related changes have not been fully established.

Differing drug responses may be approached conceptually from both a pharmacodynamic and a pharmacokinetic standpoint. The pharmacodynamic hypothesis assumes that the tissue receptor sites where drug activity occurs are more sensitive in the elderly. As a result, any given concentration of a drug reaching the tissue receptor sites will elicit a greater target organ response in an older individual than in a younger individual. Although this increased sensitivity is difficult to quantify in humans, published studies by Reidenberg, Levy, Warner, et al. (1978), Greenblatt, Allen, and Shader (1977), and Shepherd, Hewick, Moreland, and Stevenson (1977), have suggested that the elderly will exhibit a more intense pharmacological effect with such commonly used drugs as diazepam, flurazepam, or warfarin, in the absence of elevated serum concentrations. Pharmacodynamic changes in drug activity are suspected to occur with many other psychotropic drugs, but sound scientific evidence to establish this effect is lacking. Most of the documented changes in drug activity with advancing age has been linked to altered pharmacokinetic parameters (i.e., drug absorption, distribution, metabolism, and excretion). Therefore, it is important that all health practitioners understand how altered pharmacokinetics in the elderly can influence the disposition and ultimate activity of drugs in the body.

CHANGING PHARMACOKINETICS IN THE ELDERLY

Drug Absorption

The absorption of orally administered drugs is a complex process that can be influenced by a number of specific variables altered during the aging process. These variables are outlined in Table 10-1, and include gastrointestinal pH, gastric fluid volume, gastric motility, gastric emptying time, gastrointestinal blood flow, and gastrointestinal tissue changes. In addition, concomitant administration of other drugs may also alter the process of drug absorption.

Both the volume and pH of gastric fluids are altered significantly in the aging gastrointestinal tract. The incidence of hypochlorhydria or achlorhydria has been estimated by Bender (1968), Baron (1963), and Vanzant, Alverez, Eusterman, Dunn, and Berkson (1932) ten times more frequent in

Table 10-1 Factors That May Affect Drug Absorption in the Elderly

Factor	Potential Consequence
Increased gastric pH	Altered ionization of drugs
Decreased gastric fluid volume	Slowed dissolution and absorption of drugs
Decreased gastric motility	Slowed dissolution
Increased gastric emptying time	Increased destruction of acid labile drugs Delayed absorption of most drugs
Decreased mesenteric blood flow	Decreased drug absorption
Decreased number of absorbing cells	Decreased absorption of nutrients

the elderly than in younger adults, with a relatively greater incidence in women than in men. This shift to a higher pH can affect drug activity in a number of ways, since gastrointestinal pH is a primary factor that controls drug dissolution, stability, and gastric emptying. All solid oral dosage forms must initially undergo dissolution before the active drug can be absorbed. Since most drugs are classified as either weak acids or weak bases, the relative acidity or alkalinity of the gastric fluids will determine the degree of ionization of these compounds which will, in turn, determine the rate at which they will dissolve and subsequently be absorbed. Weakly acidic drugs, such as aspirin, acetaminophen, or the sulfonamides, will undergo dissolution more rapidly when the gastric fluids are less acidic, whereas weakly basic drugs, such as quinidine, codeine, or the tricyclic antidepressants, require a more acidic medium for initial dissolution. Therefore, an increase in gastric pH would most notably affect poorly soluble weakly basic drugs, or drugs that are dispersed in solid dosage forms that require a high gastric acid content for release from their dosage form.

The rate at which drugs pass from the stomach to the small intestine may influence the ultimate activity of a drug, since almost all drugs are absorbed most efficiently from the first part of the duodenum. Therefore, any delay in the passage of drugs from the stomach to the small intestine may delay and slow the rate of absorption of drugs, thereby resulting in peak blood levels that are lower than expected. In addition, drugs that are unstable in gastric acid, such as most of the penicillins, may undergo more extensive acid degradation if they remain exposed to gastric contents for a prolonged period of time. Although the rate of gastric emptying is effected by many factors that are not related to age per se, the aging process quite often is accompanied by a decline in gastric motility and tone that may prolong gastric emptying time (James, 1981; Georas & Haverback, 1969). The potential effectiveness of levodopa, a drug used to control Parkinsonism, can be used to illustrate how increasing its retention in the stomach can decrease its effectiveness. The therapeutic activity of levodopa depends to a great extent on its ability to reach the small intestine fairly rapidly, since it is sensitive to acid degradation in the stomach. Delayed gastric emptying therefore will reduce its effectiveness since it will remain in contact with gastric acids for a longer period of time. Bianchine, Calimim, Morgan, Dujovne, and Losagna (1971) demonstrated that patients whose gastric fluids were highly acidic had prolonged gastric emptying times, and subsequently had low plasma levels of levodopa. When gastric pH was elevated, gastric emptying times were increased and the plasma concentrations of levodopa rose accordingly.

Another possible basis for decreased drug absorption in the elderly may involve a decline in mesenteric blood perfusion. Blood flow to the gastrointestinal tract has been reported by Bender (1965) to decrease by as much as 40–50 percent in the elderly. Although the consequences of this reduced blood flow on drug absorption have not been clearly delineated, it appears that reduced blood perfusion to the gut may effect the rate of absorption but usually has little if any effect on the overall effectiveness of the drug. Exceptions to this rule may include drugs that are metabolized extensively on first pass through the liver, such as propranolol.

Bender (1968) also proposed that aging may be accompanied by a decline in the number of cells that are capable of facilitating drug absorption. This factor appears to be of more importance when substances that are absorbed by active transport processes are involved. Bender's studies have supported age-related decreases in the absorption of glucose, thiamine, calcium, xylose, and iron, all of which are actively absorbed. Since most drugs are absorbed primarily by simple passive diffusion, it is unlikely that drug absorption is affected by this decline.

Coadministration of other drugs may also alter drug absorption. Drugs with a high level of anticholinergic activity, such as atropine, propantheline, the tricyclic antidepressants, and most neuroleptic agents, can produce a significant decrease in gastrointestinal motility and may delay the passage of drugs from the stomach to the small intestine. Likewise, the administration of antacids with other medication can further elevate dissolution and absorption of drugs, as well as delay the passage of the stomach contents into the small intestine. Antacid therapy may also compromise drug absorption by acting as a physical barrier between the drug molecule and the mucosal cells, or may cause chemical reactions with the drug to render it more insoluble, and therefore less likely to dissolve. The familiar reaction between tetracycline derivatives and compounds containing aluminum, magnesium, calcium, bismuth, or iron is an excellent example of the latter phenomenon.

Although most of our concern has centered around the potential factors that can influence the absorption of orally administered drugs, it is important to consider how the aging process may affect drug absorption when other routes of administration are employed. Unfortunately, little if any attention has been given to the age-related differences in the absorption of drugs when given intramuscularly, subcutaneously, intravenously, sublingually, rectally, topically, or by inhalation. However, one may predict some alteration in drug absorption may occur from each of these sites, since physiological changes that occur as part of the natural aging process can affect the uptake and eventual distribution of drugs when given by any of these routes of administration.

Drug Distribution

Once the absorbed drug reaches systemic circulation, it is distributed throughout the fluids and tissues of the body in a manner than is dependent on two primary factors; the drug's inherent chemical characteristics, and the patient's physiological characteristics. These two factors operate simultaneously to allow the drug eventually to reach its site of action and evoke a pharmacological response. The extent and pattern of drug distribution are governed by several factors, including body composition, body fluid pH, plasma protein binding, tissue binding, organ blood flow, and cardiac output. Advancing age is accompanied by several gradual but dramatic changes in these factors which may influence the way drugs are distributed within the body. Novak (1972) has estimated that between the ages of 18 and 85 the proportion of body fat may increase from 18 percent to 36 percent of total body weight in men, and from 33 percent to 48 percent of total body weight in women. This change is accompanied by a decrease in lean body mass and total body water. Forbes and Reina (1970) projected that at the age of 65 the average man has 12 kg less lean body mass, and the average woman has 5 kg less, while total body water decreases 10–15 percent during this same time interval. The potential consequences of this altered body composition to changes in drug distribution depend to a great extent on the relative lipid solubility of the drug, and can be measured by observing the changes that occur in the volume of distribution (V_d) of the drug. By definition, the V_d of a drug is the hypothetical volume in which the given dose of a drug would be dispersed if its concentration in the entire body were the same as the concentration of drug in the blood. This volume will vary with each drug, and will be altered whenever there is a significant change in body composition. For example, drugs such as ethanol or digoxin are known to be confined primarily to the extracellular spaces, with very little of the total dose being taken up into body tissues. Therefore, the V_d will be small in comparison to other drugs that are able to be distributed widely to most body tissues. In the older patient, the decline in total body water can cause higher peak concentrations of these drugs if doses are based on body weight or surface area without regard to smaller extracellular fluid volume. Ewy, Kapadia, Yao, et al. (1969) demonstrated that initial levels of digoxin plus its metabolites were nearly twice as high in an elderly group of patients compared to a control group when the drug was given intravenously. These authors were able to show that the elevated peak plasma levels were a result of a smaller V_d. Vestal, McGuire, Tobin, et al. (1977) observed that peak ethanol blood levels are higher in older patients than in younger patients, and also suggested that a decrease in the V_d of ethanol was responsible for these higher blood levels. On the other hand, drugs such as diazepam, phenobarbital, and lidocaine are considered to be highly lipid soluble, and will be more extensively distributed in the elderly, particularly in the fat cells. This increase in the V_d will prolong the half-life, if clearance of the drug is unchanged. Klotz, Avant, Hoyumpa, Schenker, and Wilkinson (1975) documented dramatic increases in the V_d of diazepam in relationship to aging. These studies showed an increase in V_d of diazepam with age, which was expected from a predictable increase in the half-life of diazepam of approximately one hour each year between the ages 20 and 80. This study, as well as other reports (Greenblatt, Sellers, & Shader, 1982b; Greenblatt, Shader, & Koch-Weser, 1975), suggests that the half-life of diazepam may rise from 20 hours at the age of 20 to as much as 90 hours at the age of 80. The consequences of such a change are obvious. Excessive accumulation that may result in oversedation, disorientation, dizziness and altered mental functioning are few of the many side effects that have been observed in patients whose drug dosage had not been altered to accomodate these changes in half-life and altered distribution.

A gradual but significant fall in serum albumin concentration has been documented with aging. Misra, Loudon, and Straddon (1975) reported that plasma albumin concentration declines from a mean of 4.7 g/dl at age 25 to 3.8 g/dl at age 75. This decline may be even greater if the elderly are poorly nourished, have advanced illness, or are severely debilitated. Since most drugs establish an equlibrium in the blood between a fraction bound to plasma proteins and a free or unbound fraction, a significant decline in the number of these binding sites, which may occur with a decreased plasma albumin concentration, can alter this equilibrium to allow more free drug to be present. This shift may result in a more intense drug response than would otherwise be predicted, since the free fraction is the only portion of drug that is able to cross membranes to reach the site of pharmacological activity, or, in the case of the liver and kidney, where drug elimination can occur. Table 10-2 lists drugs that have a high affinity for plasma protein binding sites. According to Wallace, Whiting and Runcie (1976), drugs that are bound extensively to plasma proteins (such as warfarin, phenytoin, or phenylbutazone) are agents that would be most likely to elicit an exaggerated response if an increase in free drug concentration were to occur. Thus 96–98

Table 10-2 Selected Drugs Reported as Possessing a High Binding Affinity to Plasma Proteins

Drug	Percentage Bound to Plasma Proteins
Alprazolam	80
Alprenolol	85
Amitriptyline	96
Amphotericin B	90
Cefazolin	84
Chlordiazepoxide	97
Chlorothiazide	95
Chlorpromazine	96
Clindamycin	94
Clofibrate	97
Desipramine	92
Diazepam	99
Dicloxacillin	95
Digitoxin	90
Doxycycline	87
Furosemide	96
Gemfibrozil	97
Hydralazine	87
Imipramine	92
Indomethacin	90
Lorazepam	93
Notrazepam	87
Nortriptyline	95
Oxazepam	88
Phenytoin	89
Piroxicam	99
Prazosin	93
Propranolol	93
Protriptyline	92
Rifampin	89
Sulfisoxazole	90
Temazepam	96
Trazodone	90
Tolbutamide	93
Valproic acid	93
Warfarin	99

Adapted from Gilman, Goodman, and Gilman, 1980.

percent of a drug such as warfarin, under these conditions, would result in a doubling in the free fraction of the drug. As a consequence, twice as much of the drug will be available for drug action, and potential excessive anticoagulant activity and bleeding episodes may occur if the dosage is not adjusted and the patient is not carefully monitored.

The reduction in the number of available plasma protein binding sites also has potential impact on the magnitude of interactions among different drugs that involve the displacement of a drug from its binding sites in the albumin molecule by another agent, since more bound drug may be displaced due to the relative unabailability of adequate numbers of binding sites.

Metabolism

Many drugs undergo a variety of metabolic processes before being eliminated from the body. Although drug metabolism can occur in the intestinal mucosa, the plasma, and in other body fluids, the liver is the primary organ of metabolism for most drugs. Since drug metabolism is dependent on a number of variables, such as genetic predisposition, nutritional status, environmental pollution, disease states, hepatic function, and concomitant drug use, it is difficult to quantify the effect of the aging process on altered drug metabolism. Alterations in drug activity resulting from impaired drug metabolism are difficult if not impossible to predict in the elderly since none of the laboratory tests used to determine liver function can be used to assess the efficacy of hepatic metabolism. Nevertheless, a number of physiological changes occur in the liver that may have a role in altering drug metabolism and elimination. Bender (1968) observed a gradual decline in liver mass in proportion to body weight, a decrease in liver blood flow at a rate that exceeds the decline in cardiac output, and a decrease in the amount of drug metabolizing enzymes in the liver after the age of 50. He estimated the decline in liver blood flow to range from 0.3–1.5 percent each year, so that by the age of 65 hepatic blood flow is reduced by 40–50 percent in comparison to a person of 25. This decline in hepatic blood flow has been shown to effect the hepatic extraction of those drugs that are significantly cleared from the blood following oral absorption. Since hepatic extraction is the product of liver blood flow and the liver extraction ratio, drugs that are rapidly cleared by the liver are considered to have a high extraction ratio and are most effected by so-called "first pass effect." Propranolol, propoxyphene, morphine, meperidine, and lidocaine are included in this category. Extraction of these drugs may be further compromised in the presence of disease, such as congestive heart failure, which further decreases hepatic blood flow, or in combination with drugs like cimetidine, which has been reported by Feely, Wilkinson, and Wood (1981) to further compromise blood flow to the liver.

Table 10-3 Typical Pathways of Hepatic Drug Metabolism

Phase I Reactions	Phase II reactions
Hydroxylation	Glucuronide conjugation
N-dealkylation	Sulfate conjugation
Sulfoxidation	Acetylation
Nitroreduction	
Hydrolysis	

Drug metabolism can be separated into two distinct phases, as outlined in Table 10-3. Many drugs used frequently by the elderly undergo Phase I metabolism. As summarized by Lamy (1980), their metabolism may be effected to some extent by the aging process. These drugs include the tricyclic antidepressants, the oral anticoagulants, the neuroleptics, many antianxiety and sedative–hypnotic agents, and the oral hypoglycemic agents. Phase I metabolism commonly involves reactions such as oxidation, reduction, or hydroxylation, and utilizes enzyme systems such as cytochrome P-450 oxidase. These reactions occur mainly in the smooth endoplasmic reticulum of the cell, and usually lead to derivatives that are more water soluble than the original compound. Some evidence exists that elderly patients have a reduced ability to metabolize many drugs that undergo Phase I metabolism because of a reduction in liver microsomal drug metabolizing activity. Studies with antipyrine by Stevenson (1977) and O'Malley, Judge, and Crooks (1976) have reported an extended half-life and a reduced metabolic clearance in older subjects. However, other studies (Sultatos, Dvorchik, Vesell, Shand, & Bronch, 1980) demonstrate a wide variation in antipyrine metabolism and conclude that age itself is probably only a minor determinant in inhibiting antipyrine metabolism.

Phase II reactions utilize a nonmicrosomal enzyme pathway, and involve the addition of a large polar substituent to the drug molecule, thereby allowing it to be more readily excreted in the urine. The derivatives of Phase II metabolism are usually inactive. Drugs such as hydralazine, isoniazid, procainamide, and most sulfonamides undergo Phase II metabolism. Most studies conclude that age has little if any effect in altering this metabolic process.

It is important to consider that some drugs may follow a complex metabolic pathway and involve both Phase I and Phase II metabolism. An example of such complex drug metabolism is given in Figure 10-2, which involves Phase I and Phase II metabolism of diazepam.

Excretion

Renal excretion is the most important route of elimination for the majority of drugs and their metabolites. Altered renal function associated

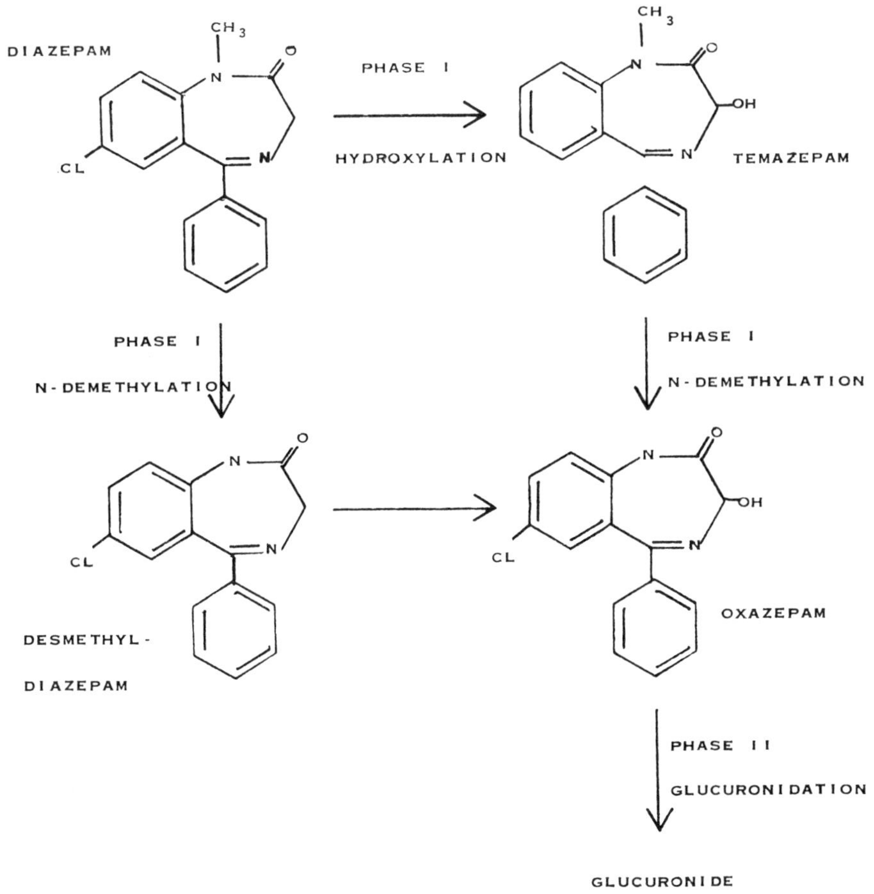

Figure 10-2. Pathway of diazepam metabolism in man. Adapted from Greenblatt and Shader, 1981.

with aging, therefore, can have important pharmacokinetic implications for many therapeutic agents. In contrast to hepatic drug metabolism, the effects of aging on renal function have been well documented in humans, and can be measured accurately by routine clinical tests. Aging produces many structural and functional changes in the human kidney. Rowe, Andres, Tobin, Norris, and Shock (1976) have reported that the glomerular filtration rate (GFR) decreases with age, so that there is a predictable decline of 35 percent in the GFR between the ages of 20 and 90.

Since lean body mass declines with age, daily endogenous creatinine production also decreases. As a result, Kampmann, Siesbaek-Nielsen, Kristensen, and Molholm-Hansen (1974) and Cockroft and Gault (1976) have shown that serum creatinine levels are not valid predictors of kidney function in the elderly, since creatinine clearance must fall to a greater extent for them before serum creatinine increases. In young patients, the GFR must fall to approximately 30 ml/min before levels of serum creatinine and blood urea nitrogen (BUN) fall into the abnormal range. In the older patient with reduced lean muscle mass, the GFR must fall to an even greater extent before serum creatinine levels rise to above the normal range. Various nomograms and formulas are available to estimate true creatinine clearance in relationship to age. A formula suggested by Cockroft and Gault that can be used to determine the patient's creatinine clearance is as follows:

$$C_{Cl} \text{ (ml/min)} = \frac{(140 - \text{age}) \times \text{body weight(kg)}}{72 \times \text{serum creatinine level}}$$

where C_{Cl} is the creatinine clearance. The result should be multiplied by 0.85 for women, and may need to be adjusted for lean body weight in obese individuals.

Since the rate of elimination of a drug determines its plasma half-life ($t_{1/2\beta}$), a decrease in renal function will prolong the drug's half-life, and may result in plasma levels of the drug that are higher than expected. This change can be particularly dangerous to the patient if the drug is excreted by the kidney in an active form, or if the drug has a low therapeutic margin of safety (e.g., digoxin) in the elderly attributed primarily to reduced renal clearance of the drug. This observation is of particular importance in terms of efficacy and safety, since the first signs of digoxin toxicity in the elderly may be manifested by confusion, disorientation, irritability, and other CNS disorders that may be mistaken for senility.

A prolongation in the elimination half-life of a drug also has an effect on the time it will take the drug to "plateau," or reach a steady state, in the plasma during maintenance therapy. For example, a drug can be considered to reach a steady state at a point in time that is between four and five times the half-life. Therefore, if a drug's half-life is reported to be 12 hours, a steady state of equilibrium will be attained in the plasma in 48 to 60 hours. At that point, plasma levels of the drug will have plateaued, and no significant increases in blood levels will occur, providing that the maintenance doses remain the same and the physiological parameters that govern half-life do not change. The plasma half-life also determines the time required to remove the drug from the body after therapy has been discontinued. As a result, impaired renal function in the elderly may result in higher, more sustained blood levels, which can result in excessive drug accumulation and toxicity. Drugs that are of particular concern include the aminoglycoside antibiotics (such as gentamicin, tobramycin, or streptomycin), the benzodiazepine derivatives that are excreted by the kidney in the active form (such as diazepam, chlordiazepoxide, flurazepam, or chlorazepate), digoxin, cimetidine, and procainamide.

PSYCHOTROPIC DRUG INTERVENTION IN THE ELDERLY

Psychiatric disorders occur more frequently in elderly patients than in younger individuals. As a result, a disproportionately greater amount of psychotropic agents are prescribed for this age group, usually by physicians not formally trained in psychiatry. Unfortunately, many conditions for which these drugs are employed are not amenable to these agents and, in fact, may have been iatrogenically produced by drugs themselves. Table 10-4 lists some of the more commonly used drugs in geriatric medicine that have been implicated as the cause of psychiatric symptoms. This table is limited to changes in mental status caused by a single drug; drug interactions have even a greater potential to cause psychiatric manifestations.

Since disease states, nutritional deficiencies, or drug therapy may precipitate psychiatric symptoms, it is important to consider these factors in addition to the patient's current mental status before attempting psychotropic drug intervention. Table 10-5 provides a guide to be used by the practitioner for screening elderly patients who are being considered as candidates for psychotropic drug therapy. In many cases, a careful review of the patient's medical problems and current drug history may uncover the source of the patient's problems. It is not uncommon to find a noticeable improvement in the patient's behavior and well-being when the number of drugs that are currently being taken is decreased and/or the dosages of the prescribed medications are decreased.

GUIDELINES FOR PSYCHOTROPIC DRUG INTERVENTION

There are four general guidelines that should be followed whenever psychotropic drug therapy is initiated. First, a therapeutic goal should be established before the drug therapy is started. For many patients, unrealistic goals may result in an unacceptably high rate of adverse drug reactions. In most cases, complete alleviation of all symptoms should not be expected, since most drugs are incapable of totally eliminating symptoms without producing harmful effects. Second, whenever possible only one drug should be added at a time to the patient's therapy. This applies also to the use of combination drug products. Initiating treatment with two or more chemotherapeutic agents separately or as a combination product not only increases the potential for drug interactions but it makes it more difficult to determine which agent may have produced beneficial or adverse effects. Third, the starting dose for most psychotropic drugs in the elderly should be 30–50 percent of the recommended starting dose for younger patients of similar size. Once the starting dose has been established, the dosage can be titrated slowly upwards (or downwards, if necessary), until the desired therapeutic endpoint has been achieved, or unacceptable side effects or adverse effects

Table 10-4 Selected Drugs Reported to Cause Psychiatric Symptoms

Drug	Reaction
Amitriptyline (Elavil; others)	Anticholinergic psychosis; see Atropine
Anticonvulsants	Tactile, visual and auditory hallucinations, delerium, agitation, depression, paranoia, confusion, aggression.
Antihistamines	Anxiety, hallucinations, delerium
Atropine and anticholinergics	Confusion, memory loss, disorientation, depersonalization, delerium, auditory and visual hallucinations, fear, paranoia
Barbiturates	See Phenobarbital
Benztropine (Cogentin)	See Atropine
Bromocriptine (Parlodel)	Mania, delusions, visual hallucinations, paranoia, aggression
Chlordiazepoxide (Librium)	See diazepam
Cimetidine (Tagemet)	Visual and auditory hallucinations, paranoia, bizzare speech, delerium, confusin, disorientation, depression
Clonazepam (Clonopin)	See diazepam
Clorazepate (Tranxene; Azene)	See diazepam
Corticosteroids (Prednisone, Hydrocortisone; others)	Mania, depression, paranoia, auditory and visual hallucinations, catatonia
Desipramine (Pertofrane)	Anticholinergic psychosis; see Atropine
Dextroamphetamine	Bizzare behavior, hallucinations, paranoia
Diazepam (Valium)	Rage, excitement, hallucinations, depression, suicidal ideation, confusion, disorientation
Diethylpropion (Tenuate)	See Dextroamphetamine
Digoxin (Lanoxin)	Nightmares, euphoria, confusion, delusions, paranoia, belligerence, visual hallucinations
Digitoxin (Crystodigin, Purodigin)	See Digoxin
Disopyramide (Norpace)	Agitation, depression, paranoia, auditory and visual hallucinations, panic
Disulfiram (Antabuse)	Delerium, depression, paranoia, auditory hallucinations
Doxepin (Sinequan, Adapin)	Anticholinergic psychosis; see Atropine
Ephedrine	Hallucinations, paranoia
Ethchlorvynol (Placidyl)	Agitation, confusion, disorientation, hallucinations, paranoia
Imipramine (Tofranil; others)	Anticholinergic psychosis; see Atropine

Table 10-4 (*continued*)

Drug	Reaction
Indomethacin (Indocin)	Depression, confusion, hallucinations, anxiety, hostility, paranoia, depersonalization
Isoniazid (INH; others)	Depression, agitation, paranoia, auditory and visual hallucinations
Levodopa (Dopar; others)	Delerium, depression, agitiation, hypomania, nightmares, night terrors, visual and auditory hallucinations, paranoia
Methyldopa (Aldomet)	Depression, hallucinations, paranoia, amnesia
Nalidixic Acid (NegGram)	Confusion, depression, excitement, visual hallucinations
Nortriptyline (Aventyl)	Anticholinergic psychosis; see Atropine
Pentazocine (Talwin)	Nightmares, hallucinations, disorientation, panic, paranoia, depersonalization, depression
Phenelzine (Nardil)	Paranoia, delusions, fear, mania, rage, aggressive behavior
Phenobarbital	Excitement, hyperactivity, visual hallucinations, depression, delerium tremens-like syndrome
Phenylephrine (Neo-Synephrine)	Depression, visual and tactile hallucinations, paranoia
Phenytoin (Dilantin; others)	See Anticonvulsants
Primidone (Mysoline)	See Anticonvulsants
Procainamide (Pronestyl)	Paranoia, hallucinations
Propoxyphene (Darvon)	Auditory hallucinations, confusion
Propranolol (Inderal)	Depression, confusion, nightmares, visual and auditory hallucinations
Protriptyline (Vivactil)	Anticholinergic psychosis; see Atropine
Rauwolfia (Serpasil; others)	Depression
Scopolamine	See Atropine
Sulindac (Clinoril)	Paranoia, rage, personality change
Tricyclic antidepressants	See Atropine
Trihexylphenidyl (Artane)	See Atropine
Trimepramine (Surmountil)	Anticholinergic psychosis; see Atropine
Zomrpirac (Zomax)	Depression, Anxiety, stupor

Adapted from Medical Letter on Drugs and Therpeutics, 1981.

Table 10-5 Factors to be Considered in Elderly Patients Before Psychotropic Drug Therapy is Initiated

- Patient History
    Are there any medical illnesses that may cause "psychiatric" symptoms?
    How long have the symptoms been present?
    Have these or similar symptoms occurred in the past?
    If so, when?
    What was the diagnosis?
    What medications, if any, were prescribed?
    It drugs were prescribed, did they help?
    Did any side effects develop?
    What current medications (prescribed and nonprescribed) are being taken?
    What nonprescription medications are being purchased?
    What is the pattern and extent of social drug use:
        If alcohol used, how much and how often is it taken?
    Does the patient smoke cigarettes?
    What is the nutritional status of the patient?

- Physical Examination
    Are there any alterations in the hepatic, renal or neurological status that could compromise drug therapy?
    What laboratory tests have been carried out to assess the patient's kidney function (has creatinine clearance been determined.?
    Has the patient's thyroid function been determined?

- Drug Interactions
    What drugs currently being taken may adversely affect or interact with the psychotropic medication under consideration?

have been eliminated. Fourth, periodic attempts should be made to taper the dose of the psychotropic drug and, for most agents, completely discontinue use. Most of these agents have established guidelines for duration of therapy and should not be continued for prolonged periods of time without good cause. A good rule to follow is *when in doubt, discontinue the medication.*

Guidelines for the common classes of psychotropic drugs are provided in the remainder of this chapter.

Sedative–Hypnotic Agents

The elderly use a disproportionately large number of drugs to induce sleep, receiving nearly 40 percent of all sedative–hypnotic prescriptions. In a recent telephone survey of the San Francisco Bay area, Miles and Dement (1978) reported that 48 percent of those over 65 admitted they took medication for sleep "every night" or "frequently." A United States Public Health Survey showed that skilled nursing facilities give almost 95 percent of their residents sedative–hypnotics, and well over 50 percent of the older patients in other institutional settings receive sleep medication on a nightly basis. Obvious misuse and abuse of sedative–hypnotics exists even though it is becoming increasingly more evident that sleep disorders in the elderly may be symptoms of many different medical or psychiatric conditions in which these drugs have no documented proof of effectiveness. In most cases, these agents can aggravate the underlying disorder and expose the individual to an increased incidence of adverse reactions that can be manifested by a deterioration in mental status and an altered functional capacity. Whenever possible, a thorough evaluation of the medical, neuropsychiatric, and psychosocial status of the elderly patient should be made before any sleep medication is prescribed. If depression is present, therapy should be aimed at treating the depressive disorder. Antidepressant therapy is the more rational drug therapy for these patients, since sedative–hypnotics are not only ineffective from a long-term standpoint, but they may further exacerbate the depressive syndrome.

If the patient's sleep disorder is a result of organic brain disease or other psychotic disorder, these agents are again not only ineffective but may increase the patient's agitation and disorientation. Antipsychotic therapy may be more appropriate in these patients. For many other elderly insomniacs whose condition stems from other medically related problems, such as arthritis or other conditions that cause chronic pain or discomfort, sedative–hypnotics may lead to nightly dependence and increase the risk of misuse or abuse.

There are many drugs marketed specifically for the treatment of insomnia and other sleep disorders. These agents include the classical barbiturates such as pentobarbital (Nembutal), the non-barbiturate sedative–hypnotics such as glutethimide (Doriden), methaqualone (Quaalude, Parest), or chloral hydrate (Noctec, Somnos), and the benzodiazepine derivatives such as flurazepam (Dalmane), temazepam (Restoril), and triazolam (Halcion). Occasionally antihistamines such as diphenhydramine (Benadryl) have been employed to induce drowsiness, but a report (Thompson, Moran, & Nies, 1983) has suggested that they are associated with a higher risk of delerium in the elderly than the benzodiazepines. Antihistamines are most frequently found in nonprescription sleep aids.

Fortunately, reports from the United States Public Health Service state that the use of the barbiturates and the non-barbiturate sedative–hypnotic agents has declined dramatically since 1971. Table 10-6 outlines the disadvantages associated with the use of these agents. With the possible exception of chloral hydrate, they have no place in the treatment of sleep disorders in the elderly.

Since the benzodiazepines are the most frequently prescribed sedative–hypnotics, it is important to have a thorough understanding of the differences that exist among these agents, and the drawbacks and limitations

Table 10-6 Disadvantages of the Barbiturate and Non-Barbiturate Sedative–Hypnotic Agents

• Significant alteration of sleep stages

• Rapid development of tolerance and withdrawal phenomena

• Low margin of safety

• Potential for drug interactions by stimulation of hepatic microsomal enzyme systems

• Rapid loss of therapeutic effectiveness

that should be considered when one is used. All benzodiazepines, including those used as antianxiety agents (such as diazepam or lorazepam) will, in low doses, produce an anxiolytic effect and, in larger doses, produce sleep. However, only flurazepam, temazepam, and triazolam are marketed specifically for the treatment of insomnia. More importantly, it should be recognized that adverse drug reactions can occur with all of these agents, and may include confusion, disinhibition, aggression, ataxia, hallucinations, depression, restlessness, rage, and altered cognitive and psychomotor function. In the elderly, these adverse reactions appear to be more likely to occur with drugs that are inherently long-acting, and whose active drug or metabolites are excreted by the kidney. An analysis of the data in Table 10-7 reveals significant differences between the pharmacokinetic profiles of these compounds, which should be considered whenever any of these agents is employed.

Table 10-7 Pharmacokinetic Profiles of the Benzodiazepines Used to Treat Insomnia

Drug	Active Components	Rate of Absorption or Appearance	Rate of Elimination (Half-Life Range)
Flurazepam (Dalmane)	Hydroxyflurazepam	Rapid	Rapid (8–12 h)
	Flurazepam aldehyde	Rapid	Rapid (8–12 h)
	Desalkylflurazepam	Slow	Slow (40–200 h)
Temazepam (Restoril)	Temazepam	Slow	Intermediate (10–20 h)
Triazolam (Halcion)	Triazolam	Intermediate	Rapid (1.5–5 h)

Adapted from Greenblatt, Divoll, Abernethy, and Shader, 1982.

Flurazepam is the most frequently prescribed sleep medication in the United States and, according to Solomon, White, Parron, and Mendelson (1979), accounts for nearly 60 percent of all sedative–hypnotic prescriptions written. The drug has a complex pharmacokinetic profile in that it must be converted to active metabolites in order to produce a pharmacological response. Two metabolites, hydroxy-flurazepam and flurazepam aldehyde, appear rapidly and are responsible for initiating sleep, are rapidly eliminated from the body, and are not likely to produce accumulation on repeated usage. The third metabolite, desalkylflurazepam, appears more slowly and, according to Greenblatt, Allen, & Shader (1977), exhibits a half-life of between 50 and 100 hours that may be extended to 300 hours in elderly males. Kaplan, deSilva, Jack, et al. (1973) reported plasma levels of this metabolite at steady state to be as much as 4–6 times the levels obtained after the first dose. As a result, continued usage of flurazepam on a nightly basis may result in excessive daytime sedation and may interfere with cognitive functioning and psychomotor performance. The potential for flurazepam to produce adverse effects has been clearly related to the aging process and the size of the dose administered. In a well-documented study involving over 2500 in-patients, Greenblatt, Allen, and Shader (1977) reported that only 2 percent of those 70 years of age or older experienced adverse effects with flurazepam if the dosage was less than 15 mg/day. The incidence of adverse reactions to flurazepam in this age group, however, rose to 39 percent when doses of 30 mg or more of the drug were administered. Nearly all adverse drug reactions documented in this study involved drowsiness, confusion, or ataxia, and were reversed when the drug was discontinued. Such side effects can be particularly dangerous to the elderly patient, since accidents, including falls, occur more frequently, and the confused or disoriented state may be mistaken for senility or dementia and antipsychotic medication may be added to the patient's drug therapy. Based on the results of this study, there appears to be little justification to using a bedtime dose of flurazepam of more than 15 mg and, considering its prolonged half-life, it may be appropriate to dose flurazepam every other day or every third day.

Temazepam is a minor metabolite of diazepam and is classified as a benzodiazepine with an intermediate half-life of between 10–20 hours. Unlike flurazepam, it has been shown by Schwartz (1981), to be converted to inactive metabolites by the liver. Therefore, drug accumulation is much less of a problem when this drug is given in equivalent doses and intervals. However, studies by Divoll, Greenblatt, Harmatz, and Shader (1977) indicate that the absorption and onset of activity is slow, with peak blood levels occurring from 1.5–2 hours after administration. Therefore, it has been suggested that when temazepam is used it should be given an hour or two before bedtime to accomodate the slower absorption. Roth, Piccione, Salis, et al. (1979) reported fewer hangover effects with temazepam compared to flurazepam, and had significantly fewer deleterious effects on performance. However, a report by Cook (1980) documents a cumulative effect with temazepam, although total accumulation was not of the magnitude as produced by flurazepam.

Triazolam is classified as an ultra-short sedative–hypnotic and has a half-life of 1.5–5 hours. It has been shown by Chatwin and Jonns (1977) and Wang and Stockdale (1973) to have an intermediate onset of action, and will generally shorten the latency to sleep onset and reduce the number of nocturnal awakenings in most individuals. Metzler, Ko, Royer, et al. (1977) reported little or no accumulation of triazolam or its metabolites in the plasma after several consecutive days of therapy. Although most studies report that triazolam is equal to or better than flurazepam, Morgan and Oswald (1982) have observed "rebound insomnia" with this agent, and have reported a potential for increased daytime anxiety when triazolam is employed. Further investigations concerning these potential problems need to be carried out.

Regardless of which sedative–hypnotic is used, drug therapy should be considered only as an adjunct to the treatment of the sleep disorder, and should not be used for an indefinite period of time. Most studies recommend a period of no longer than two weeks at doses that are as low as possible. With flurazepam and temazepam, nighttime doses should not exceed 15 mg, and with triazolam, doses should be no greater than 0.25 mg. In addition, a careful evaluation of the patient's drug history is essential since the incidence of CNS toxicity to these agents is greatly increased if other CNS depressants, such as alcohol, are consumed.

Antianxiety Agents

The most frequently prescribed anxiolytic agents are the benzodiazepines. They have largely replaced drugs such as phenobarbital and meprobamate in controlling excessive anxiety. These latter two agents are particularly dangerous in the elderly, since they rapidly produce tolerance, have a low therapy to toxicity ratio, and they may stimulate the metabolism of other currently administered drugs. As a result, the risk to benefit ratio is not acceptable, and there is no justification for use as antianxiety agents in the elderly.

All benzodiazepines have similar activity. They reduce anxiety and promote sleep, have anticonvulsant properties, and are capable of producing muscle relaxation. They also have the potential, when used indiscriminately or incorrectly, for producing excessive sedation, ataxia, confusion, disorientation, forgetfulness, paradoxical excitement and aggressiveness, and depression. Despite these similarities, there are differences in the pharmacokinetics of these compounds that should be considered when selecting these agents for use in the elderly. Table 10-8 lists the benzodiazepines currently available and classifies them according to their metabolic rate.

Table 10-8 Pharmacokinetic Comparison of the Benzodiazepines Used as Antianxiety Agents.

Class I Benzodiazepines Metabolized to Active Compounds		
Drug	Active Metabolite	Elimination Half-life
Chlordiazepoxide (Librium)	Desmethylchlordiazepoxide Demoxepam Desmethyldiazepam	— 28–63 hr 50–99 hr
Clorazepate (Tranxene, Azene)	Desmethyldiazepam	50–99 hr
Diazepam	Desmethyldiazepam	50–99 hr
Halazepam (Paxipam)	Desmethyldiazepam	50–99 hr
Prazepam (Verstran)	Desmethylidazepam	50–99 hr

Class II Benzodiazepines Metabolized to Inactive Compounds	
Drug	Elimination Half-life
Lorazepam (Ativan)	8–24 hr
Oxazepam (serax)	7–25 hr

Class III Benzodiazepines With Small Amounts of Active Metabolites	
Drug	Elimination Half-life
Alprazolam (Xanax)	12–15 hr

Adapted from Breimer, Jochemsen, and von Albert, 1980.

Depending on the specific compound, aging has been shown to alter the distribution and elimination of these agents at various rates. Klotz, Avant, Hoyumpa, Schenker, and Wilkinson (1975) reported a prolongation in the half-life of diazepam of approximately one hour each year of age past 20, so that the projected half-life in an 80 year old person may be as high as 90 hours. Roberts, Wilkinson, Branch, and Schenker (1978) also documented an increased half-life of chlordiazepoxide with age, increasing from seven hours at age 20 to over 40 years at age 80. Since most of the benzodiazepines

Table 10-9 Hazards of the Long-Acting Benzodiazepines in the Elderly

• Accumulation of long-lived active metabolites when used on consecutive or alternate days

• An increasing likelihood of adverse drug reactions with increasing age of the patient

• A greater likelihood of adverse drug reactions in patients with diminished renal function

• Additive and possible synergic effects with other CNS depressants including alcohol

• Decreased daytime visual–motor coordination on repeated doses

• Potential for drug dependence with continued use

• Increased respiratory depression

are metabolized to the same metabolites as diazepam, a similar extension in their half-life could be expected. As a result of these changes in drug half-life, there is a greater likelihood for excessive accumulation and, correspondingly, a greater potential for intoxication if the dosage is not adjusted. Table 10-9 lists the hazards that are likely to result when long-acting benzodiazepines are used in the elderly. Since blood levels will continue to increase until a steady state is reached, the therapeutic as well as toxic effects may not be fully evident until days after therapy had been started. Likewise, clinical effects may persist for days after the drug is discontinued, and adverse reactions will be resolved more slowly. The steady state is the point in time at which blood levels will plateau, so that continued dosages of the drug on a daily basis will not result in a further elevation of plasma levels. This point in time can be estimated by multiplying the half-life by four or five; if a drug has a half-life of 24 hours, steady state will be reached in four or five days. With drugs like diazepam, after steady state has been reached blood levels will not be substantially altered if the daily dose is a divided or a single dose. Therefore, one has to seriously question the wisdom of prescribing drugs with long half-lives for three or four doses a day. On the other hand, Shull, Wilkinson, Johnson, and Schenker (1976), Greenblatt, Shader, and Koch-Weser (1975), and Kraus, Desmond, Marshall, et al. (1978) reported no significant prolongation in the half-life of lorazepam or oxazepam, since their metabolites are inactive. As a result, these derivatives may be a more logical choice for use in elderly patients when anxiolytic therapy is indicated, and are more logically prescribed for two or three doses a day.

Regardless of the specific benzodiazepine that is chosen, appropriate use of these agents requires a careful evaluation of the patient before the drug is given. Depressed patients, or those with mild or subclinical dementia, may experience a worsening of their condition which may not be recognized as drug-induced by the physician or nurse. In addition, a complete drug history should be attained so that drug interactions can be avoided. It is particularly important to identify other drugs that have the ability to cause drowsiness or sedation, since excessive CNS depression may result. It is not uncommon to find elderly patients taking a long-acting benzodiazepine such as diazepam during the day and a sedative–hypnotic such as flurazepam at bedtime for sleep. This type of combination therapy is not only irrational but is destined to result in excessive sedation and other manifestations of intoxication and should be condemned. Although the benzodiazepines are not likely to alter the metabolism of other drugs, certain agents may affect the metabolism of some of the benzodiazepines. Cimetidine (Tagamet®) has been shown by Klotz and Reimann (1980) and by Desmond, Patwardhan, Schenker, et al. (1980) to delay the clearance of diazepam and chlordiazepoxide, which can result in excessive drug accumulation and increased CNS toxicity. On the other hand, Patwardhan, Yarborough, Desmont, et al. (1980) demonstrated that the benzodiazepines that are converted to inactive metabolites are spared of this interaction.

Antidepressant Agents

Depression is one of the most common disorders in the elderly effecting at least one in ten individuals in this age group at any given time. Bressler (1982) reports that more than half of these older individuals experience their first episode after the age of 60. Many disease states, such as hyper- or hypothyroidism, Parkinson's disease, nutritional deficiencies, pneumonia, or cancer, can precipitate or aggravate depression. Likewise, many different drugs, such as reserpine, propranolol, levodopa, the sedative–hypnotics, or corticosteroids, have been associated with precipitating or aggravating depression. Their role in the depressive syndrome should be ruled out before therapy is instituted.

When drug intervention is needed, a specific agent is usually chosen from the list of antidepressants found in Table 10-10. These agents differ quite widely in their anticholinergic and sedative potentials, and initial selection should be based on the patient's need for sedation and ability to tolerate anticholinergic side effects. Excessive anticholinergic activity may be responsible for a number of potentially serious side effects, such as tachycardia, arrhythmias, blurred vision, urinary retention, orthostatic hypotention, and sexual dysfunction. In addition, an anticholinergic psychosis may be precipitated that can produce delerium, disorientation, memory loss, hallucinations, and paranoia, which may not be attributed to the

Table 10-10 Profiles of the Commonly used Antidepressants

Drug	Sedation	Anticholinergic	Cardiovascular
Amitriptyline (Elavil; others)	High	High	High
Doxepin (Adapin, Sinequan)	High	High	Moderate
Nortriptyline (Aventyl)	Moderate	Moderate	High
Imipramine (Tofranil; others)	Moderate	Moderate	High
Desipramine (Pertofrane)	Low	Low	Moderate
Protriptyline (Vivactil)	Very low	Moderate	High
Trimipramine (Surmountil)	High	High	High
Amoxapine (Asendin)	Moderate	Moderate	Low
Maprotiline (Ludiomil)	Moderate	Moderate	Moderate
Trazodone (Desyrel)	Moderate	Very Low	Very Low

antidepressant medication. Attention should also be given to the anticholinergic activity that may exist with other current medications. It is not uncommon to find neuroleptic agents, such as thioridazine, or antiparkinson drugs, such as benztropine, also being administered. These drugs possess substantial anticholinergic activity, and their combination with an antidepressant may result in excessive anticholinergic activity.

Initial dosing of antidepressant medication should be at a level between a third to a half the usual recommended adult dose, and should be given in divided doses, since the elderly typically exhibit a decreased tolerance to the side effects of these agents. The dose is adjusted gradually, based on the patient's clinical response and the appearance of side effects. It must be emphasized that significant variability between patients exists in terms of the size of the doses and the patients' responses. A study by Montgomery, Braithwaite, and Crammer (1977) revealed that optimum nortriptyline blood levels were achieved in patients with daily doses that ranged from 25 mg/day to 150 mg/day. The study underscores the need to individualize dosing regimens for each patient, and may explain why tricyclic antidepressant therapy is frequently unsuccessful in the elderly and why so many adverse reactions occur with this class of drugs. Once the therapeutic dose has been achieved, it is advantageous to administer the entire daily dose once a day, preferably at bedtime, if the patient is able to tolerate it.

Antidepressant therapy should be carried out for at least four weeks before therapy with another antidepressant is considered. If at least two antidepressants from Table 10-8 have been tried unsuccessfully, the use of a monoamine oxidase inhibitor such as tranylcypromine may be considered. However, strict attention must be given to the types of food consumed by the patient who is given a monoamine oxidase inhibitor, since foods containing significant amounts of tyramine may interact with the antidepressant and result in a significant elevation in blood pressure that may end in a hypertensive crisis. In addition, monoamine oxidase inhibitors inhibit the metabolism of drugs that undergo Phase I metabolism in the liver, so it is important to obtain a thorough medication history, including all prescription and nonprescription drugs.

Antipsychotic Agents

Antipsychotic or neuroleptic drugs are employed to treat various psychotic states such as schizophrenia, manic–depressive disorders, and psychoses associated with organic brain syndrome. They are not to be considered "tranquilizers" to be used to sedate non-psychotic patients, nor should they be employed as sleep medication to treat insomnia that is not based on a psychiatric disorder. Yet these drugs are commonly prescribed for the elderly, and represent the most frequently prescribed class of drugs for institutionalized psychiatric patients. In a survey of geriatric patients in 12 Veteran's Administration hospitals, Prien, Haber, and Caffey (1975) reported that antipsychotic agents were prescribed four times more frequently than any other psychoactive agent. The most common neuroleptic agent prescribed for these patients was thioridazine, accounting for 40 percent of the antipsychotic prescriptions. Altman, Evenson, Sletten, and Cho (1972) reported similar findings in a similar study. Ray, Federspiel, and Schaffner (1980), in a review of prescriptions in nursing homes, found that 43 percent of the residents received antipsychotic medication. The most frequent combination was an antipsychotic and a sedative–hypnotic (usually thoridazine and flurazepam), followed by anxiolytic and sedative–hypnotic (diazepam and chloral hydrate). The most frequently prescribed antipsychotics were thioridazine, chlorpromazine, and haloperidol. In Sweden a study of drug-induced deaths not attributed to intentional suicide (Bottinger, Norlander, Strandberg, & Westerholm, 1977) reported that psychotropic agents were primarily involved in nine percent of the reported deaths, and that age-related adverse drug reactions to this class of agents rose from 2–3/100,000 at age 55 to 15–16/100,000 at age 70. This apparent increase in adverse drug reactions to the neuroleptics may be attributed to both pharmacodynamic changes at the receptor sites in the CNS as well as altered drug distribution, metabolism, and excretion, as discussed previously in this chapter. Yet there have been only a few published reports that have

Table 10-11 Side Effect Profiles of Selected Antipsychotic Agents

Drug	Sedation	EPS*	Anticholinergic	Cardiovascular
Chlorpromazine (Thorazine)	HIgh	Moderate	Moderate	High
Thioridazine (Mellaril)	High	Low	High	High
Loxapine (Loxitane)	Moderate	High	Low	Moderate
Fluphenazine (Prolixin; Permitil)	Low	High	Low	Low
Haloperidol	Very low	Very high	Very low	Very low

* Extrapyramidal symptoms.

investigated the relationship of age to increased variability in the response to these agents.

Table 10-11 outlines the side effect profiles of a representative group of neuroleptic agents. From this table it is obvious that adverse reactions to these drugs will be based to a large extent on the individual drug that is employed. It should be pointed out that studies such as those conducted by Altman and associates, and Tsuang, Lu, Stotsky, and Cole (1971), did not demonstrate any consistent differences in the clinical efficacy with any specific agent in treating organic brain syndrome or schizophrenia. Likewise, all neuroleptics can produce similar adverse effects, but these will vary, sometimes considerably, in their degree and prevalence. The most widely documented adverse reactions from antipsychotic therapy are the extrapyramidal side effects that include acute dystonias, akathesia, perioral tremor, pseudo-Parkinsonism, and tardive dyskinesia. These occur most frequently with haloperidol therapy. In a study by Ayd (1979) extrapyramidal symptoms were seen in 50 percent of the patients between the ages of 60 and 80 who were treated with neuroleptics. Although antiparkinson drugs, such as benztropine or trihexiphenidyl, are employed in the treatment of these extrapyramidal reactions, their use is being seriously challenged in the elderly, since these drugs have substantial anticholinergic activity and may produce psychotic reactions themselves. Additional reports (Parker, 1981) have associated the combination of neuroleptic drugs and antiparkinson agents with an increased likelihood of tardive dyskinesia. If antiparkinson agents are to be employed they should be added to the patient's therapy only when the extrapyramidal symptoms appear. The only exception to this rule is when the long-acting injection of fluphenazine (Prolixin Decanoate®) is used. Antiparkinson agents can be stopped without the recurrence of extrapyramidal symptoms in 90 percent of the patients after three months of therapy.

When antipsychotic drug therapy is initiated in the geriatric patient, it should be recognized that there is no standard dose for the use of neuroleptic agents. As a rule, the older patient should be started on a small, divided dose to assess the presence and significance of adverse reactions. Initial doses that are too high may be likely to precipitate acute dystonias or excessive sedation. If the initial dose is well-tolerated, then the dose can be doubled at approximately three day intervals, until there is a partial improvement in the condition or the patient exhibits significant adverse reactions. If the patient's target symptoms do not begin to respond to drug therapy after three weeks, either the dose should be increased or the patient should be switched to another neuroleptic. If large doses are ineffective, suspect either noncompliance by the patient, or an incorrect diagnosis. Since most of these agents have long half-lives (24 hours or longer for most), one dose a day can be implemented once the patient's dose has been stabilized. Administration at bedtime is preferable in most patients, since they may sleep through the peak anticholinergic and sedative effects. Although it is common to find patients taking more than one antipsychotic agent at the same time, there is no substantial evidence to support the contention that two or more neuroleptics are more efficacious than one, or are safer than an adequate dose of a single drug. Careful attention needs to be given to potential drug interactions with other medications. In particular, drugs such as the antidepressants or the antiparkinson agents have anticholinergic activities and may enhance anticholinergic induced side effects, such as dry mouth, urinary retention, blurred vision, or constipation. Excessive anticholinergic activity may also precipitate an anticholinergic psychosis as described previously in this chapter. In addition to the common adverse reactions, such as the sedative, anticholinergic, extrapyramidal, and cardiovascular effects that may be seen with these agents, it is important to recognize that some agents have unique reactions that need to be taken into consideration. Antipsychotics that have significant sedative activity also appear to have a significant potential to produce orthostatic hypotension, which can lead to an increased incidence of dizziness, unsteadiness, fainting, and falls. Blood pressure measurements in both the supine and standing position should, therefore, be taken regularly during the initial stages of treatment. Other drug-induced side effects include an increased sensitivity to ultraviolet light, a disruption in normal body temperature control that may result in hypo- or hyperthermia depending on the surrounding temperature, and the development of pigmentary retinopathy which may alter color vision and decrease visual acuity. In addition, blood dyscrasias, endocrine changes, and lowering of the seizure threshold have been reported to occur more frequently with these agents in the elderly population. More detailed reviews of the side effects and adverse drug reactions to the neuroleptics are provided by Baldessarini (1980) and Inoue (1979). In summary, the following points should be considered whenever antipsychotic drug therapy is initiated in the elderly.

1. A comprehensive patient history should be obtained prior to initiating therapy.
2. Become familiar with the incidence of side effects of the antipsychotic being considered.
3. Use only one antipsychotic at a time.
4. The choice of antipsychotic agent should be based on the patient's needs, general health, and/or other medical problems.
5. If large doses are ineffective, suspect noncompliance by patient, or a missed diagnosis.
6. Whenever possible, administer once a day.
7. Use antiparkinson drugs only when extrapyramidal symptoms appear. Discontinue as soon as possible.
8. Consider potential drug interactions that may increase either the possibility of sedation or anticholinergic side effects.
9. Emphasize compliance.
10. Attempt to decrease the dose or discontinue the medication at regular intervals.

SUMMARY

Drug therapy must be approached cautiously in the aging patient because there are so many variables that can alter the way drugs behave in the body. We are just beginning to gain an understanding of the complexity of drug activity in the older patient, and how the aging process can alter drug activity and response. Although models or guidelines have been proposed to quantify the rate or extent of changes in pharmacokinetics and pharmacodynamics that occur with age, other studies force us to recognize the potential problems that may result from these age-related changes, and thus allow us to avoid many of the pitfalls in drug therapy that have gone undetected in the past. In particular, psychotropic drug therapy in the elderly must be evaluated very critically. The following points should be kept in mind when these agents are employed.

1. A therapeutic plan with realistic goals and expectations should be developed before drug therapy is initiated.
2. Appropriate laboratory tests should be carried out whenever possible before drug therapy is started; a creatinine clearance test is essential.
3. The number of drugs prescribed should be kept at a minimum, and the regimen of doses should be as simple as possible.
4. A complete medication profile should be obtained and maintained to minimize drug interactions.
5. Doses should be smaller than the recommended adult doses; older patients are more sensitive to the therapeutic as well as toxic effects of these agents.

6. Adverse drug reactions are more prevalent in the elderly and may be more difficult to recognize.

REFERENCES

Altman, H., Evenson, R.C., Sletten, I.W., & Cho, D.W. (1972). Patterns of psychotropic drug prescriptions in four midwestern state hospitals. *Current Therapeutic Research, 14*, 667–672.

Ayd, F.J. (1979). A survey of drug-induced extrapyramidal reactions. *JAMA, 175*, 1054–1060.

Baldessarini, R.J. (1980). Drugs in the treatment of psychiatric disorders. *In* A.G. Gilman, L.S. Goodman, & A. Gilman (Eds.), *The pharmacological basis of therapeutics* (6th ed.) (pp. 391–418). New York: Macmillan.

Baron, L.H. (1963). Studies of basal and peak acid output with an augmented histamine test. *Gut, 4*, 136–141.

Bender, A.D. (1968). Effect of age on intestinal absorption: Implications for drug absorption in the elderly. *Journal of the American Geriatrics Society, 16*, 1331–1339.

Bender, A.D. (1965). The effect of increasing age on the distribution of peripheral blood flow in man. *Journal of the American Geriatrics Society 13*, 192–198.

Bender, A.D., Post, A., Meier, J.P., et al. (1973). Plasma protein binding of drugs as a function of age in adult human subjets. *Journal of Pharmaceutical Sciences, 64*, 1711–1713.

Bianchine, J.R., Calimim, L.R., Morgan, J.P., Dujovne, C.A., & Lasagna, L. (1971). Metabolism and absorption of L-3,4 dihydroxyphenalinine in patients with Parkinson's disease. *Annals of the New York Academy of Sciences, 179*, 126–139.

Bressler, R. (1982). Antidepressant therapy. In K.A. Conrad & R. Bressler (Eds.), *Drug therapy for the elderly* (pp. 295-315). St Louis: C.V. Mosby Co.

Bottinger, L.E., Nordlander, M., Strandberg, I., & Westerholm, B. (1974). Deaths from drugs. An analysis of drug-induced deaths reported to the Swedish Adverse Drug Reaction Committee during a five-year period (1966-1970). *Journal of Clinical Pharmacology, 14*, 401–407.

Breimer, D.D., Jochemsen, R., & vonAlbert, H.H. (1980). Pharmacokinetics of benzodiazepines. *Arzneim Forsch, 30*, 875–881.

Chatwin, J.C., & Johns, W.L. (1977). Triazolam: An effective hypnotic in general practice. *Current Therapeutic Research, 21*, 207–214.

Christopher, L.J. (1978). Patterns of prescribing in general practice. In H.F. Woods (Ed.), Topics in therapeutics (6th ed.) (pp. 1–14). London: Pitman Books, Limited.

Cockroft, D.W., & Gault, M.H. (1976). Prediction of creatinine clearance from serum creatinine. *Nephron, 16*, 31–41.

Committee on Ways and Means, United States House of Representatives (1971). *Basic facts of health industry* (p. 29). Washington, DC: Government Printing Office.

Cook, P. (1980). Change in benzodiazepine drug activity with aging. In A.N. Exton-Smith (Ed.), *Current trends in therapeutics in the elderly* (pp. 23–32). Oxford: Medical Education Services, Ltd.

Desmond, P.V., Patwardhan, R.V., Schenker, S., et al. (1980). Cimetidine impairs the elimination of chlordiazepoxide (librium) in man. *Annals of Internal Medicine*, *93*, 266–268.

Divoll, M., Greenblatt, D.S., Harmatz, J.S., & Shader, R.I. (1977). Effect of age and gender on disposition of temazepam. *British Journal of Clinical Pharmacology*, *8*, 23–95.

Drugs that cause psychiatric symptoms (1981). *The Medical Letter on Drugs and Therapeutics*, *23*, 9–12.

Ewy, G.A., Kapadia, G.G., Yao, L., et al. (1969). Digoxin metabolism in the elderly. *Circulation*, *39*, 449–453.

Feely, J., Wilkinson, G.R., & Wood, A.J.J. (1981). Reduction of liver blood flow and propranolol metabolism by cimetidine. *New England Journal of Medicine*, *304*, 692–695.

Forbes, G.B., & Reina, J.C. (1970). Adult lean body mass declines with age: Some longitudinal observations. *Metabolism*, *19*, 653–663.

Georas, M.C., & Haverback, B.J. (1969). The aging gastrointestinal tract. *American Journal of Surgery*, *117*, 881–892.

Gilman, A.G., Goodman, L.S., & Gilman, A. (1980). *The pharmacological basis of therapeutics* (6th ed.) (pp. 1684–1739). New York: Macmillan, 1980.

Greenblatt, D.J., Allen, M.D., & Shader, R.I. (1977). Toxicity of high-dose flurazepam in the elderly. *Clinical Pharmacology and Therapeutics*, *21*, 355–361.

Greenblatt, D.J., Divoll, M., Abernethy, D.R., & Shader, R.I. (1982a). Benzodiazepine hypnotics: Kinetics and therapeutic options. *Sleep*, *5*, 518–527.

Greenblatt, D.J., Sellers, T.M., & Shader, R.I. (1982b). Drug disposition in old age. *New England Journal of Medicine*, *306*, 1081–1088.

Greenblatt, D.J., & Shader, R.I. (1981). Pharmacokinetics in old age: Principles and problems of assessment. In L.F. Jarvik (Ed.), *Clinical pharmacology and the aged patient*, (pp. 27–46). New York: Raven Press.

Greenblatt, D.J., Shader, R.I., & Koch-Weser, J. (1975). Pharmacokinetics in clinical medicine: Oxazepam versus other benzodiazepines. *Diseases of the Nervous System*, *36*, (section 5), 6–13.

Hurwitz, N. (1969). Predisposing factors in adverse reactions to drugs. *British Medical Journal*, *1*, 536–539.

Inoue, F. (1979). Adverse reactions of antipsychotic drugs. *Drug Intelligence and Clinical Pharmacy*, *13*, 192–208.

James, O.F. (1981). The absorption and distribution of drugs in old age. In F.I. Caird & J.G. Evans (Eds.), *Advanced Geriatric Medicine I*, (pp. 3–13). London: Pitman Books, Limited.

Kampmann, J., Siesbaek-Nielsen, K., Kristensen, M., & Molholm-Hansen, J. (1974). Rapid evaluation of creatinine clearance. *Acta Medical Scandinavica*, *196*, 517–520.

Kaplan, S.A., de Silva, J.A.F., Jack, M.L., et al. (1973). Blood level profile in man following chronic oral administration of flurazepam hydrochloride. *Journal of Pharmaceutical Sciences*, *62*, 1932–1935.

Kiernan, P.J., & Issacs, J.B. (1981). Use of drugs by the elderly. *Journal of the Society of Medicine*, *74*, 196–200.

Klotz, U., Avant, G.R., Hoyumpa, A., Schenker, S., & Wilkinson, G.R. (1975). The effects of age and liver disease on the disposition and elimination of diazepam in adult man. *Journal of Clinical Investigation*, 55, 347–359.

Klotz, U., & Reimann, I. (1980). Delayed clearance of diazepam due to cimetidine. *New England Journal of Medicine*, 302, 1012–1014.

Kovar, M. (1977). Health of the elderly and use of health services. *Public Health Reports*, 92, 9–19.

Kraus, J.W., Desmond, P.V., Marshall, J.P., et al. (1978). Effects of aging and liver disease on the disposition of lorazepam. *Clinical Pharmacology and Therapeutics*, 24, 411–419.

Lamy, P.P. (1980). *Prescribing for the elderly* (pp. 249–292). Littleton, MA: PSG Publishing.

Lamy, P.P., & Vestal, R.E. (1976). Drug prescribing for the elderly. *Hospital Practice*, 11, 111–114.

Metzler, C.M., Ko, H., Royer, M.E., et al. (1977). Bioavailability and pharmacokinetics or orally administered triazolam in normal subjects. *Clinical Pharmacology and Therapeutics*, 21, 11–12.

Miles, L.E., & Dement, W. (1978). *Sleep and aging*. Paper prepared for the National Institute on Aging Conference on Sleep and Aging.

Misra, D.P., Loudon, J.M., & Staddon, G.E. (1975). Albumin metabolism in elderly patients. *Journal of Gerontology*, 30, 304–306.

Montgomery, S., Braithwaite, R.A., & Crammer, J.L. (1977). Routine nortriptyline levels in the treatment of depression. *British Medical Journal*, 3, 166–167.

Morgan, K., & Oswald, I. (1982). Anxiety caused by a short-term hypnotic. *British Medical Journal*, 282, 942.

Nies, A., Robinson, D.S., Friedman, M.J., et al. (1977). Relationship between age and tricyclic antidepressant levels. *American Journal of Psychiatry*, 134, 790–793.

Norris, A.H., Lundy, I., & Shock, N.W. (1963). Trends in elected indices of body composition in men between the ages of 30 and 80 years. *Annals of the New York Academy of Science*, 110, 623–639.

Novak, L.P. (1972). Aging, total body potassium, fat free mass and cell mass in males and females between the ages 18 and 85 years. *Journal of Gerontology*, 27, 438–443.

O'Malley, K., Judge, T.G., & Crooks, J. (1976). Geriatric clinical pharmacology and therapeutics. In G.S. Avery (Ed.), *Drug treatment: Principles and practice of clinical pharmacology and therapeutics* (pp. 123–142). Sydney: ADIS Press.

Ouslander, J.G. (1981). Drug therapy in the elderly. *Annals of Internal Medicine*, 95, 711–722.

Parker, J.D. (1981). Adverse effects of antiparinsonian drugs. *Drugs*, 21, 341–353.

Patwardhan, R.V., Yarborough, G.W., Desmond, P.V., et al. (1980). Cinetidine spares the glucuronidation of lorazepam and oxazepam. *Gastroenerology*, 79, 912–916.

Prien, R.F., Haber, P.A., & Caffey, E.M. (1975). The use of psychoactive drugs in elderly patients with psychiatric disorders: Survey conducted in twelve Veterans Administration hospitals. *Journal of the American Geriatrics Society*, 23, 104–112.

Ramsay, L., & Tucker, G.T. (1981). Drugs and the elderly. *British Medical Journal*, 282, 125–127.

Ray, W.A., Federspiel, C.F., & Schaffner, W. (1980). A study of antipsychotic drug use in nursing homes. Epidemiologic evidence suggesting misuse. *American Journal of Public Health, 70*, 385–491.

Reidenberg, M.M., Levy, M., Warner, H. et al. (1978). Relationship between diazepam dose, plasma level, age, and central nervous system depression. *Clinical Pharmacology and Therapeutics, 23*, 371–374.

Riley, G.A. (1977). How aging influences drug therapy. *US Pharmacist, 2*, 29–43.

Roberts, R.K., Wilkinson, G.R., Branch, R.A., Schenker, S. (1978). Effects of age and parenchymal liver disease on the disposition and elimination of chlordiazepoxide (librium). *Gastroenterology, 75*, 479-485.

Roth, T., Piccione, P., Salis, P., et al. (1979). Effects of temazepam, flurazepam and quinalbarbitone on sleep: Psychomotor and cognitive function. *British Journal of Clinical Pharmacology, 8*, 47–54S.

Rowe, J.W., Andres, R., Tobin J.D., Norris, A.H., & Shock, N.W. (1976). The effect of age on creatinine clearance in man: A cross-sectional and longitudinal study. *Journal of Gerontology, 31*, 155–163.

Schwartz, H.J. (1981). Pharmacokinetics and metabolism of temazepam in man and several animal species. *British Journal of Clinical Pharmacology, 8*, 23–29S.

Shepherd, A.M., Hewick, D.S., Moreland, I.A., & Stevenson, I.H. (1977). Age as a determinant of sensitivity to warfarin. *British Journal of Clinical Pharmacology, 4*, 315–320.

Shull, H.J., Jr., Wilkinson, G.R., Johnson, R., & Schenker, S. (1976). Normal disposition of oxazepam in acute viral hepatitis and cirrhosis. *Annals of Internal Medicine, 84*, 420–425.

Smith, J.W., Seidl, L.G., & Cluff, L.E. (1977). Studies on the epidemiology of adverse drug reactions. *Annals of Internal Medicine, 65*, 629–640.

Solomon, F., White, C.C., Parron, D.L., & Mendelson, W.B. (1979). Sleeping pills, insomnia and medical practice. *New England Journal of Medicine, 300*, 803–808.

Stevenson, I.H. (1977). Factors influencing antipyrine elimination. *British Journal of Clinical Pharmacology, 4*, 261–266.

Sultatos, L.G., Dvorchik, B.H., Vesell, E.S., Shand, D.G., & Branch, R.A. (1980). Further observations on relationships between antipyrine half-life, clearance and volume of distribution: An appraisal of alternative kinetic parameters used to assess the elimination of antipyrine. *Clinical Pharmacokinetics, 5*, 263–273.

Thompson, T.L., Moran, M.G., & Nies, A.S. (1983). Psychotropic drug use in the elderly: Part. I *New England Journal of Medicine, 308*, 134–138.

Triggs, T.J., & Nation, R.L. (1975). Pharmacokinetics in the aged: A review. *Journal of Pharmacokinetics and Biopharmacy, 3*, 387–418.

Tsuang, M.M., Lu, L.M., Stotsky, B.A., & Cole, J.O. (1971). Haloperidol versus thioridazine for hospitalized psychogeriatric patients: Double-blind study. *Journal of the Geriatrics Society, 19*, 593–600.

Vanzant, G., Alvorez, W.C., Eusterman, G.B., Dunn, H.L., & Berkson, J. (1932). The normal range of gastric acidity from youth to old age: An analysis of 3,746 records. *Archives of Internal Medicine, 49*, 345–349.

Vestal, R.E. (1978). Drug use in the elderly: A review of problems and special considerations. *Drugs, 16*, 358–362.

Vestal, R.E., McGuire, E.A., Tobin, J.D., et al. (1977). Aging and ethanol metabolism. *Clinical Pharmacology and Therapeutics, 21*, 343–354.

Wallace, S., Whiting, B., & Runcie, J. (1976). Factors affecting drug binding in plasma of elderly patients. *British Journal of Clinical Pharmacology*, *3*, 327–330.

Wang, R.I.H. and Stockdale, S.L. (1973). The hypnotic efficacy of triazolam. *Journal of International Medical Research*, *1*, 600–607.

Williamson, J., & Chapin, J.M. (1980). Adverse reactions to prescribed drugs in the elderly: A multicentre investigation. *Age and Ageing*, *9*, 73–80.

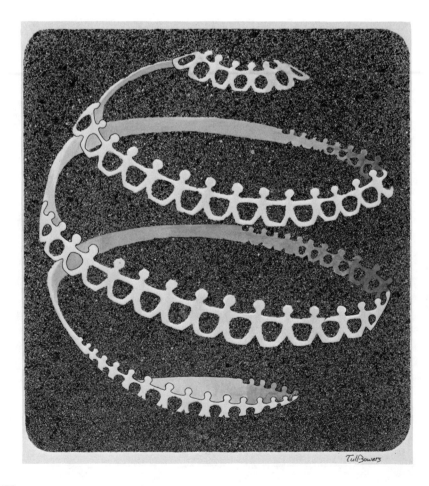

Chapter 11

Sociotherapy

The problems of old age are often erroneously attributed to older people instead of to the gaps that have been created between the needs of those people and the approaches taken to address their needs. The emergence of a new gerontocracy which attempts to define its own destiny is one manifestation of society's failure to meet either individual or group needs.

This chapter examines the array of programs that have developed in recent years, and the processes that influence whether or not available services are utilized. The spectrum of services has broadened to include almost all aspects of life for the elderly, yet problems still exist in many areas, defining the nature of work that remains to be done. Inequities in home health care services, self-help or advocacy activity, limited outreach programs, and the role government will come to play, are discussed as issues reflecting the concern and commitment of society to the aged and as guidelines for future endeavor.

SOCIAL INITIATIVE

The success of sociotherapeutic interventions depends in large measure on the efficacy of psychotherapeutic interventions; educational programs that debunk myth and stereotype, research discoveries that illuminate and dispell murky assumptions, and programs for the media that alter attitudes of young and old alike.

In their study of psychological distress among community elderly, Abrahams and Patterson (1978-1979) found that the ability of older adults to take social initiatives (i.e., to organize a varied daily activity pattern and maintain relationships beyond the household) was closely associated with psychological health. Social initiative depended upon several factors:

- Whether mental health services were available but unused because they did not reach out to the elderly
- Whether psychologically distressed elderly who were isolated, or living alone in restricted family units, lacked adequate outside contact
- Whether information and referral services available in centers for the elderly were utilized
- Whether the high-risk elderly (those poorly educated, physically impaired, or living in deteriorated neighborhoods) were able to develop relationships beyond the household.

Ethnicity bore little relationship to psychological impairment, but past histories of psychopathology accounted for the cumulative disadvantageous effects of dependency and poor coping ability seen throughout the remainder of life. Abrahams and Patterson recommend the establishment of community support systems not only for the elderly but the middle-aged as well to link older adults to outreach programs and prevent the crippling effects of isolation before the combined effects of physical, mental, and social deficit result in irreparable damage. Simply providing social services cannot suffice to meet the needs of older adults if awareness and access to programs is impeded.

NAVIGATING THE HUMAN SERVICE SYSTEM

Our human service system is difficult to navigate, and the older adult is not usually equipped either physically or emotionally to traverse the pitfalls without support. Despite the formidable array of services and programs already in existence, many gaps in an otherwise comprehensive network do appear, often leaving the older adult uncertain as to where and how to get help. One of the major sources of support in recent years has been expansion of social or socializing networks for the elderly, which provide new opportunities and structures for meaningful social involvement of older adults as a group. Cohen (1980) cites five socializing networks that aid navigation.

1. Longevity allows the development of four or five generation families, increasing the adult's base of familial social involvement and support.
2. Volunteerism and focused involvement in civic affairs (even holding political office) is a reflection of the growing new gerontocracy.
3. Recreational and athletic opportunities for the elderly are proliferating.
4. Educational pursuits through continuing education programs offer opportunity for dynamic exchanges between generations in classrooms.

5. Post-retirement opportunities enable individuals to assume second and even third careers.

The key to successful utilization of available community resources lies in knowing that they exist and finding the means by which to gain access. Communities sometimes offer outreach satellite programs in neighborhood centers, while others provide the services of paid outreach workers. Youth groups of various ages have volunteered to seek out, identify, and link with the appropriate group those isolated elders who would otherwise not be served. Television and radio programs provide valuable informational links and many offer call-in services that explain where and how help can be obtained.

DAY CARE SERVICES

The day care concept has provided an invaluable support base for preventative health services in many European countries, and has been recognized as an equally valuable component of health care in this country as well. Individuals with some degree of nonincapacitating mental or physical illness are able to remain within the community if supportive services are provided. Care may be available for 8 hours a day, 5 days a week, with transportation and meal service provided. The program is subdivided according to the targeted health care, socialization, mental health, or psychosocial needs of older adults, and the agency's defined mission. Intensive, restorative ambulatory care is made available for adults who do not require 24 hour institutional care but are unable to maintain full-time independent living. In other programs time-limited or long-term restorative services provide care for older adults whose high-risk health status warrants closer supervision and monitoring. The focus of still other agencies is on socialization needs of primarily frail yet ambulant adults who require a safe environment, supervised activities, rest, and at least one nutritious meal daily. Despite differences, in each instance the goal is to keep older adults out of institutions.

SENIOR CENTERS

Senior centers are frequently confused with social day care centers, but they differ in that they provide social activities for elderly persons who do not require any custodial care. The expansion of senior centers was accelerated by funds from the Older Americans Act, Title V, that made possible the construction of facilities and development of programs throughout this country. As of 1975 more than 5,000 senior centers were in operation, and the number keeps increasing. The diversity of programs and services provided by the centers is determined locally, and is determined by the local philosophy of normal aging, wellness, and preventative mental health. Lowy (1980) cites the typical services provided:

- Information
- Referral and brief direct services
- Casework assessment
- Some counseling
- Service coordination
- Home health care
- Brief medical and psychosocial evaluation
- Financial management
- Legal and protective guardianship service
- Transportation or escort services
- Cash for emergencies
- Meal service
- Volunteer services

FOOD AND NUTRITION PROGRAMS

The Comprehensive Services Amendments to the Older Americans Act of 1972 established a national program that has successfully addressed two problems simultaneously; inadequate nutrition and social isolation. Under this congregate meal program, nutritionally sound meals are served in strategically located centers, such as school cafeterias, churches, community centers, or public and private facilities. With emphasis on the impovershed and isolated aged, congregate meal programs served well over 200 million meals in all 50 states during the first five years of their opperation. Meals-on-Wheels programs also provide a vital link between the outside world and the homebound elderly. Most Meals-on-Wheels programs have remained small in scale and are operated mainly by voluntary organizations. Food stamps, which may be purchased at less than face value, can be used to pay for Meals-on-Wheels services, or may be used for direct foodstore purchases.

TRANSPORTATION

Access to services is a critical need of the older adult. Many elderly cannot afford the cost of private automobiles or public transit systems, and others are reluctant to face the uncertainties of driving or mass transit subway and bus rides. Despite a national policy mandating public access to mass transportation facilities, Lowy (1980) states that no systematic implementation of the national policy on accessibility has been established.

Community volunteerism is still the principal source of transportation, with various agencies and groups providing special buses and vans, coordinated through a central information exchange, as part of senior citizen mobile service programs.

HOMEMAKER SERVICES

Homemaker services usually include services aimed at preserving and maintaining the family environment threatened by disruptive effects of illness or social maladjustment. The major functions of the homemaker service include laundry, shopping, and meal preparation. Home health aides may also provide light housekeeping services in addition to taking vital signs, bathing the patient, and assisting with physical therapy needs. The term *homemaker–home health aide* is often used to refer to this type of health care professional. The goal of both services is the improvement in quality of life for the elderly, particularly those facing potential institution-alization. The number of homemaker–home health aide programs has increased significantly in recent years. In some instances service is provided by private corporations that subcontract with agencies. Present estimates place the number of available programs nationwide at only ten percent of projected need, and this critical deficit has remained uncorrected.

HOME HEALTH CARE

Home health care programs also remain seriously jeopardized by insufficient number of physicians in addition to other deficiencies (Kart, Metress, & Metress, 1978). Some of these are:

- Rising medical costs that make health care too expensive for all but the most affluent elderly.
- Inadequate Medicare coverage that denies service to millions of older adults ineligible for Medicaid yet unable to pay out-of-pocket expenses.
- Fragmented health and medical services.
- Increases in the number of more serious illnesses, multiple health problems, and chronic disorders requiring recurrent medical care.
- Lack of a good health care system that recognizes the value of deeper human resources.

Nursing remains the major health profession that provides home health care, through public health and visiting nurse agencies. The projected burden for nurses in the years ahead is expected to well exceed all available personnel resources. In rural settings, community nurses often provide the only direct contact the elderly person has with the community. Hospital-based programs have been in short supply, and have tended to emphasize short-term intensive needs of patients rather than long-range needs. Although the number of home health agencies increased during the early 1970s, more recent estimates reveal a decline in number. In addition to the number of programs, the distribution of services is often poor and in some regions of the country no services are available. Efforts to include greater emphasis on home health services are increasing, but no major changes are likely to occur prior to passage of national health insurance legislation.

EDUCATION

The thrust of educational programs has been directed to the learning needs of older adults, and the knowledge deficits of health care providers. The elderly have been known to accept stereotypes regarding old age even more than younger persons, and the concerted efforts of Gray Panthers, Green Thumb, Foster Grandparents, National Caucus of the Black Aged, American Association of Retired Persons, and National Retired Teachers Association have been directed to challenging stereotyped images and improving well-being through learning-oriented promotional programs.

Today's elderly have less formal education than any other group in society, with approximately 20 percent listed as functionally illiterate. Colleges, universities, adult and continuing education programs, and neighborhood civic associations have attempted to offset this by establishing educational programs that provide instrumental life skills (to improve day-to-day functioning) and expressive skills (to enrich life through creative self-expression). At this time more than 500 institutions of higher education are offering courses designed to meet the needs of the elderly.

The need for continued education of health professionals is evident in the number of gerontological programs offering specialized training in the physical, social, or psychological needs of the elderly. Educational programs have enabled care givers to find various ways in which patients' learned helplessness can be prevented. Fuller (1978) reports on several successful attempts at restoring freedom of choice to patients. Solomon (1982) also reports on the success of three- and four-day professional seminars, using film, videotape, experiential exercises, and group discussions, in demythologizing and educating health workers to the positive, growth-oriented potential of senescence.

PEER COUNSELING

Peer assistance programs have emerged from the growing self-help movement. The assistance offered by one aged person to another may involve housing, telephone checks, meals, or health care. More formalized programs have adopted the same concept of peer help in establishing counseling assistance. The reluctance of professionally trained therapists to provide counseling services to the elderly resulted, according to Garfinkel (1975), from the notion that older adults simply did not talk much.

Peer counseling programs have captured wide attention because they not only dispel several myths of aging but also demonstrate the ability of the older adult to provide psychological help for himself and others. Peer counseling programs typically require only a few weeks of intensive theoretical and clinical training, in which a lay "helper" learns to apply knowledge and skills to the "helpee's" problem. Personal resources that may be used to improve coping strategies and resolve problems are identified. The peer counselor is often sought by the helpee because of recognized similarities, as a generalist who is knowledgeable about human relations and community resources, as a specialist who has experienced and achieved successful adjustment through adaptation strategies, and as a life veteran whose cognizance of aging's physical, social, and psychological dilemmas reflects experiential savvy and commonality.

ADVOCACY

The recent mobilization to political awareness of older adults has resulted in the emergence of a group identity, one with substantial potential for initiating social change. The effect of improved morale, quality of life, and outlook of individuals and groups is quite encouraging. While the intent of advocacy groups is the direct involvement of older adults on behalf of themselves in the administration of services, a secondary gain, of even greater importance, is their sense of independent self-maintenance. There is no viable alternative to the sense of personal and collective potential that membership in an advocacy group brings. Butler and Lewis (1977) argue strongly in support of advocacy as the principal means of bringing about needed social change to protect the rights of the older adult. They decry all romantic illusions associated with past attempts to work within the system. They suggest that "to work at all on the problems of the elderly, as with all groups that have suffered or are suffering injustices, one must be willing to be angry and outraged, depressed and despairing; but always ready and spoiling for a struggle."

CONSUMERISM

As consciousness of the elderly within our society rises, the likelihood of meeting their mental health needs is increased by rather dynamic developments in program and policy formulation. The key factor in the emergence of mental health programs is a rise in consumerism, the growing concern of the public over the quality of public services and products. Cohen (1980) sagely reminds us that as the stereotypes of old age are demythologized and clarified, problems that can be resolved by intervention become apparent.

A careful reexamination of former expectations follows in the wake of growing dissatisfaction of consumers in general, and the elderly in particular. Former acceptance of negative changes in mental health during senescence are increasingly being challenged. Cohen perceives an "inverse relationship between how well old age is perceived and valued and how much society will take for granted about it." Much of what society has taken for granted is under careful scrutiny. He cites as one of the more positive signs for the future of America's elderly their recent integration in intergenerational families, now widely depicted in television scenarios that test new social ideas and capture the fantasy life of our culture.

Health professionals would be well-advised to acknowledge the rise in consumer distrust of health care practices by demanding realistic media depictions of how effective complete health care delivery can be for the elderly. Neither nursing nor medicine has attempted to refute the public's perception of health care abuses by requesting equal time from the media, and this glaring omission leaves unabated many consumer concerns.

RIGHT TO TREATMENT

The right of the older adult to treatment is an issue of legal and ethical concern. Landmark decisions, such as that of *Donaldson v. O'Connor* (1976), clearly affirmed the right of the incarcerated individual to treatment while confined within the institution. Yet countless numbers of elderly patients are involuntarily confined within settings that provide no more than custodial care. The next logical step is focusing public attention on the illegality of institutionalization under these circumstances.

The relocation of elderly patients from psychiatric treatment resources to nursing homes does not excuse the nursing home from responsibility for treatment, even if it is devoid of mental health treatment services. Although the political climate favoring patients' rights is still being legitimatized through court rulings, the question of whether the nursing home can justify not treating mental disturbances on the grounds that resources are not at their disposal is not likely to be ruled upon favorably, given existing legal precedents.

Lawton (1982) states that treatment is a rare phenomenon. While data showed that 70 percent of institutions for the elderly in the United States offered structured activity programs (arts and crafts), only 19 percent of the residents participated; similarly, while 19 percent of institutions offered residents opportunities for work, only 4 percent of residents actually worked. In a study of 44 nursing homes in which residents' activity was directly observed, in only two percent of some 28,000 separate observations was any nursing or medical treatment being given. Social behavior occurred in 17 percent of the observations, and in more than 50 percent no categorizable behavior was seen.

THE ROLE OF GOVERNMENT

Government is heavily involved in health care delivery in the United States and yet its precise role has not been determined. Jonas, Banta, and Enright (1977), raise several pertinent questions.

What proportion of payment for health services will be public money? Who shall plan how funds are used? Who shall assure quality? The tangled net of programs, with multiple jurisdictions and interests, leading to overlapping coverage for many people and lack of coverage for others, presents a major difficulty. But a more serious problem is defining the relation between government and the private sector. What we need is not a government takeover, but a rational division of labor between the public and private sectors; a cooperative effort aimed at benefitting the citizenry rather than aggrandizing either sector.

The lack of a precisely determined governmental role is nowhere more evident than in the payment social security benefits. With the system still in jeopardy of bankruptcy, compromise plans to tax benefits, although designed to increase revenues, will be met with strong resistance. Also, benefits may be cut, or supplemental cost-of-living adjustments will not be made. Rising social security costs and widespread doubts about the system's future have led to a withdrawal from participation in growing numbers of schools, churches, hospitals, and municipal groups. Continued withdrawal in preference to less expensive private pension plans is estimated to cost some $18 billion in revenue. As of fall 1982, 456 hospitals and 399 nonprofit agencies had submitted notification of withdrawal intent.

Federally funded programs in health care delivery and research have proliferated in recent decades, yet often without adequate attention of the government to monitoring procedures. The absence of quality assurance requirements or adequate quality monitoring clauses are keenly felt in these programs.

Findings of congressional and special senatorial studies have repeatedly pointed out the lack of a coherent national manpower training policy, but until very recently little had been done. The amount and quality of training in geriatric mental health remains low. Attention must be given to the training of providers who spend most of their time in direct service to aged patients. Cohen (1980) recommends striking a balance between the development of training centers and the provision of individual fellowships, between career development and continuing education, between clinical training and research training, and between training for professionals and education for the elderly and their families.

RESEARCH

Although service and psychosocial research should continue to receive emphasis, special attention should be given also to research on mental illness among older adults, since its prevalence is disproportionately high, and activity in this area has been scant.

Aging is known to significantly influence numerous physiological variables, and because the diagnosis of disease depends upon defined differences between normal and abnormal states, it is essential to define age-adjusted criteria for clinically relevant variables. Cross-sectional studies are frequently misinterpreted. Rowe (1977) points out that subjects over age 75 represent a sample of biologically superior survivors from a cohort that has experienced at least a 75 percent mortality. If the variable under study is related to survival, either because it is a risk factor or has a protective effect, a cross-sectional effect will suggest age-related differences that do not exist. These methodological obstacles can be avoided with use of prospective, longitudinal study designs, in which subjects are followed over a period of time and the rate of change of each variable is calculated for each group followed.

Many research questions await investigation. Too little is known about the effects of loss in one system on the performance other systems. For example, how and why are lipofuscin accumulations, plaque formation, or neurofibrillary proliferation related to neocortical deterioration in certain instances, but not in others?

AN INTERNATIONAL PERSPECTIVE

The response of professionals and nonprofessionals alike to the needs of America's aged has been heartening and commendable, but a great deal more remains to be done. In other developed countries, industrialization, urbanization, increased gross national product, an aging population, and increased social expenditures, have modified the function of the aged in the economy as well as social relationships. In these relatively more affluent countries, the wage economy has slowly displaced older adults from traditionally held roles. The pathway selected by developing nations, however, still implys a substantial commitment to the family as a basic unit of society, a commitment that Morris and Leavitt (1982) believe is reflected in reality; the family remains a major resource for care of the aged. They also cite public policies that suggest that in developing nations a tendency to follow in the steps of developed countries is very much in evidence; that the basis of public health care is the provision of a national insurance system, even if it is limited to a thin segment of the population. Many questions are being raised in developing nations as to whether the limited resources available for social services are best directed in patterns that inherited from developed countries; institutional care followed by income maintenance and health care, followed by transfer of major care responsibilities to formal and professional institutions, with only token home-care support services. Other options include government support of nonprofessional, noninstitutional programs of a mutual aid.

Economic growth does promise and deliver industrial (rather than collective, family, or group) freedom. As a result of a flexible wage and cash economy, each person has a right to independently conduct his life as he chooses. However, Morris and Leavitt raise several ethical choices that provide a fitting end to this examination of aging and mental health. Freedom's obligations are often obscured by its euphoria. The euphoria that accompanies such opportunity often obscures the obligations that personal freedom entails.

Such obligations are often considered transferable to social services on an open-ended basis. In developed countries the steady reduction in personal disposable income that has taken place over the last few decades has led to a reaction against the tax-supported social provisions that sometimes conceal a neglect of the helpless populations. The borderline between freedom and selfishness has become obscured. The central moral questions that will underlie the evolution of personal social services in developing nations deal with the proper balance between personal rights and obligations and governmental obligations.

SUMMARY

Social initiatives to intervention with the elderly depend in large part upon the success of prior psychotherapeutic interventions. The ability of the individual to utilize the human service system is greatly facilitated by information and referral services that clearly indicate where, how, and by what means contact with agencies can be made. A growing network of community outreach programs establishes a vital support base, particularly for the inexperienced client.

An ever-increasing spectrum of services—day care, senior center, nutrition, transportation, homemaking, and home health services—although still inadequate in sheer numbers, do provide optimism and encouragement.

Education and peer counseling programs reflect the desire of individuals of all ages to learn their way behind the mythology of old age and strike out in laudable acts of self-determination.

Advocacy programs and rising interest consumer protection alert us to the responsibility we all share in protecting and asserting ourselves in an increasingly complex world. The role of government in the lives of older Americans is still undecided. Given the speed and ease of global interaction and communication, this may no longer be a uniquely American problem, but one inexorably linked to all world populations. The only "real" question that remains is the location of the borderline between freedom and selfishness.

REFERENCES

Abrahams, R. & Patterson, R. (1978-1979). Psychological distress among the community elderly: Prevalence, Characteristics, and implications for service. *International Journal of Aging and Human Development, 9*(1), 1–17.
Assaulted from all sides. (1983, January 31). *Time,* p. 28.
Butler, R. & Lewis, M. (1977). *Aging and mental health* (p. 278). St. Louis: C. V. Mosby Company.
Cohen, G. (1980). Prospects for mental health and aging. In J. Birren & R. Sloane (Eds.), *Handbook of mental health and aging* (p. 278). Englewood Cliffs, NJ: Prentice-Hall, Inc.
Fuller, S. (1978). Inhibiting helplessness in elderly people. *Journal of Gerontology Nursing, 4*(4) 18–21.
Garfinkel, R. (1975). The reluctant therapist. *Gerontology, 15*(2), 136–137.
Jonas, S., Banta, D., & Enright, M. (1977). Government in the health care delivery system. In S. Jonas (Ed.), *Health care delivery in the united states* (pp. 325–326). New York: Springer Publishing Company.
Kart, C., Metress, E., & Metress, J. (1978). *Aging and health.* Menlo Park, CA: Addison-Wesley Publishing Company.
Lawton, M. (1982). Environments and living arrangements. In R. Binstock, W. Chow, & J. Schulz (Eds.), *International perspectives on aging: Population and policy challenges* (pp. 159–182). New York: United Nations Fund for Population Activities.
Lowy, L. (1980). Mental health services in the community. In J. Birren & R. Sloane (Eds.), *Handbook of mental health and aging* (pp. 827–853). Englewood Cliffs, NJ: Prentice-Hall, Inc.
Morris, R. & Leavitt, T. (1982). Issues of social service policy. In R. Binstock, W. Chow, & J. Schulz (Eds.), *International perspectives on aging: Population and policy challenges* (p. 215). New York: United Nations Fund for Populations Activities.
Rowe, J. (1977). Clinical research on aging: Strategies and directions. *New England Journal of Medicine, 297*(24), 1332–1336.
Solomon, K. (1982). Social antecedents of learned helplessness in the health care setting. *Gerontology, 22*(3): 282–287.
Watzlawick, P., Weakland, J., & Fisch, R. (1974). *Change. Principles of problem formation and problem resolution* (p. 159). New York: W. W. Norton and Company.

Appendix:

Laboratory Values

Laboratory values for the elderly are included here to provide assistance in clarifying clinical departures from normal standards, and to provide a reference tool for psychiatric nurses. When compared to standards derived from younger subjects, many questions arise about whether deviations from those standards are actually a result of normal age-related physiological change, of which too little is known, or a consequence of some disease process.

The laboratory values reflect the study of a large population of healthy adults. Subjects were drawn from various settings, including nursing homes as well as private dwellings. Studies that reported findings for institutionalized subjects were omitted, with the exception of Maekawa's (1976) examination of home versus institutionalized subjects, which was included for comparative purposes. A wide age range is represented, and sample sizes vary considerably. Data are presented in compiled, abridged form to aid the reader in differentiating deviations in value and age.

Examination of hematological values (Tables A–C) reveals generally lower values and wider ranges than those of young adults. Sex related differences appear to be less than those in younger subjects, and men show slightly higher limits. The greater female RBC range (Table A) may be a function of institutionalization, but both that range and the range for females at home remain within normal limits. White cell and differential counts both fall within normal limits but, the range has been extended higher and lower. An appreciable range extension is found for platelet count, but findings from various studies have yielded conflicting interpretations that may be due in

---

All standard normal values reported are from Davidshohn and Henry, 1974.
Reported ranges are within two standard deviations (95%) of normal values.
In all tables, N indicates the sample size.

part to differences in measurement technique. Most researchers currently believe that there is little change in platelet count with age.

Hayes & Stinson (1976) reported a steady increase in erythrocyte sedimentation rate values (Table D) with age, and a similar decrease in percentage of subjects falling within normal limits. Albumin values (Table E) were found to lower slightly with age, while total bilirubin ranges fell within normal limits except for men over 70 (Table F). Blood urea nitrogen (Table G) mean values reported by Werner (1970) show an increase with age for both sexes, particularly for women, and these data corroborate similar earlier findings.

Calcium values (Table H) declined for men, but remained essentially unchanged for women. Cholesterol values, which are known to rise with age, were found by Cutler (1970) (Table I) to be in excess of standard normal limits, but he and others agree that many healthy elderly subjects frequently exceed them. A slight but steady increase with age in creatinine (Table J) was found for both men and women, while a noteworthy decline in creatinine clearance was found for men (Table K) (Rowe, 1976) Data for women were unavailable. Ranges for subjects in all age groups were shown to exceed standard normal values for fasting glucose, but the greatest excess occured among subjects beyond the sixth decade (Table L). Findings for inorganic phosphorus (Table M) have tended to be equivocal and often conflicting, but results of Wilding, Rollason, and Robinson (1972) indicate an increase in inorganic phosphorus with age, and a broadening of ranges as well. Older women show a tendency toward higher values.

A slight increase in potassium (Table N) and an equally slight decline in total protein (Table O) are apparent with age. Data from Wilding's study suggest only little fluctuation in sodium level with age, in contrast to other investigations which have reported greater variance in mean value and range (Table P). Uric acid levels show higher values for men at all ages, but an even greater increase for women with aging (Table Q).

Data for glucose tolerance support the widely held assumption of an increase in postprandial glucose values with age. All older subjects in Andres and Tobin's (1977) review exceeded normal limits at the one-hour post-challenge period (Table R). The authors caution us that the values presented indicate mean values and not the upper limits of normality.

Initial sex related differences in mean alkaline phosphatase values (Table S) are reduced with age. Older subjects have been known to demonstrate marked increases in alkaline phosphatase, increases which may approach 150 percent of standard normal values.

Values for lactate dehydrogenase (Table T) reveal increases with age but no evidence of difference according to sex. Serum glutamic oxalacetic transamenase values for men show little change with age, but values for women show a steady increase, though both groups remain well within normal limits (Table U) The paucity of available data on serum glutamic pyruvic transamenase and age precludes any possible conclusion. Findings (Conconi, et al, (1963) reveal an obvious decline with age, but one that continues to remain within normal limits. Data on serum creatine phosphokinase values have not been readily available, but some researchers studying small samples have reported an absence of any significant change with age.

Urinalysis findings in healthy aged subjects (Table V) may not reveal dramatic evidence of age-related change, but minimal dilution capacity and maximal concentration capacity have been shown to decrease with age. Changes in the number of functioning nephrons and glomerular filtration rate increase the relative solute load to which the aging kidney must respond, and limits its ability to maintain homeostasis at extremes of hydration or dehydration.

A review of the data suggests that patterns of increase and decrease in value often seem to exhibit radical change at or near the sixth or seventh decades. Women seem to exhibit greater variation in values with age. Reasons for these phenomena are presently unclear, and it remains for further studies to provide answers. Interpretation of laboratory findings such as these is difficult for several reasons. Normative data for this age group are only now being compiled. Consequently, judgements can only be made cautiously. Comparisons are inevitably made with previously standardized, well-known groups, a process which frequently tends to compell researchers to draw inappropriate conclusions from their new data. This must be guarded against. As new means are established for older age groups, normal departures from those means appear quite natural, resulting in new interpretations of variance. Addition of new data increases the possible normal variance, and may place in jeopardy a subject who happens to fall at either extreme end of the distribution by labeling their value abnormal. They may be fully within their own normal range.

Table A Red Blood Cell Count

Sex	Age	N	Mean (10^6/mm^3)	Range (10^6/mm^3)
M*	60+	110	4.14	3.1–5.2
F*	60+	152	3.93	2.9–4.0
M**	60+	50	4.60	3.4–5.8
F**	60+	45	4.33	3.4–5.3

Adapted from Maekawa, 1976.
* Reside at home.
** Reside in institution.
Standard Normal Values: M—4.6–6.2, F—4.2–5.4.

Table B Hemoglobin and Hematocrit Values of Men Aged 65–91

Substance	Sex	Age	N	Mean	Range
Hemoglobin*	M	65–91	47	15.0 (gm/dl)	14.0–16.0
Hematocrit**	M	65–91	47	44.0 (%)	38.0–50.0

Adapted from Libow, 1963.
* Standard Normal Values: M—13.5–18.0, F—12.0–16.0.
** Standard Normal Values: M—40.0–54.0, F—38.0–47.0.

Table C Total WBC, Differential, and Platelet Count of Subjects Aged 60–95

	Sex	Age	N	Mean	Range
Total WBC (mm^3)*	M	60–95	50	7,730	4,250–16,000
	F	60–95	50	6,497	3,150–10,350
Differential (%)					
Basophils	M	60–95	50	1.1	0.0–4.0
	F	60–95	50	1.0	0.0–3.0
Eosinophils	M	60–95	50	4.4	0.0–9.0
	F	60–95	50	4.7	0.0–17.0
Bands or stabs	M	60–95	50	1.4	0.0–5.0
	F	60–95	50	1.8	0.0–8.0
Polys or segs	M	60–95	50	59.1	28.0–86.0
	F	60–95	50	55.6	28.0–75.0
Lymphocytes	M	60–95	50	23.5	4.0–46.0
	F	60–95	50	27.7	11.0–62.0
Monocytes	M	60–95	50	10.4	4.0–26.0
	F	60–95	50	9.1	2.0–19.0
Platelet Count (#/cm^3)**					
	M	60–95	50	732,000	255,000–1,392,000
	F	60–95	50	781,000	330,000–1,430,000
	M/F	60–89	94		70,266–172,000

Adapted from Shapleigh, Mayes, and Moore, 1952.
* Standard Normal Values = M—4,500–11,000/mm^3, F—4,500–11,000/mm^3.
** Standard Normal Values: M/F—150,000–400,000/mm^3. Dameshek Method Normal Values: M/F—400,000–800,000/mm^3.

Table D Erythrocyte Sedimentation Rate

Age	N (Both Sexes)	Mean (mm/hr)	Range	Percentage Within Normal Range
20–29	23	8.8	1–20	100
30–39	26	11.7	2–32	88
40–49	24	14.8	2–30	79
50–59	25	15.0	3–35	76
60–69	32	19.3	6–40	53
70–79	22	22.7	4–50	54
80+	17	26.8	14–54	53

Adapted from Hayes and Stinson, 1976.
Standard Normal Values: M under age 50 < 15 mm/hr, over age 50 < 20 mm/hr, F under age 50 < 20 mm/hr, over age 50 < 30 mm/hr.

Table E Age, Sex and Serum Albumin Level

Sex	Age	N	Mean (gm/dl)	Range
M	20–39	1529	3.99	3.2–4.8
M	40–59	2009	3.87	3.0–4.7
M	60–79	382	3.67	2.9–4.4
F	20–39	1943	3.68	3.0–4.4
F	40–59	2355	3.64	2.9–4.4
F	60–79	590	3.64	3.0–4.3

Adapted from Cutler, 1970.
Standard Normal Value: M—3.2–4.5 gm/dl, F—3.2–4.5 gm/dl (salt fractionation).

Table F Age, Sex and Total Bilirubin Level

Sex	Age	N	Mean (mg/dl)	Range
M	20–39	817	0.64	0.0–1.3
M	40–59	2380	0.62	0.0–1.2
M	60–79	520	0.64	0.0–1.7
F	20–39	265	0.53	0.0–1.1
F	40–59	561	0.53	0.0–1.1
F	60–79	768	0.50	0.0–1.0

Adapted from Wilding, Rollason, and Robinson, 1972.
Standard Normal Value: M—0.1–1.2 mg/dl, F—0.1–1.2 mg/dl.

Table G Blood Urea Nitrogen Mean Values by Age and Sex

Sex*	Age	Mean (mg/dl)
M	20–29	17.5
M	30–39	17.0
M	40–49	17.9
M	50–59	18.9
M	60–69	20.4
M	70–79	18.1
F	20–29	13.8
F	30–39	14.2
F	40–49	16.3
F	50–59	16.9
F	60–69	18.9
F	70–79	18.9

Adapted from Werner, 1972.
* Total sample size combining both sexes, was greater than 3000.
Standard Normal Value: M—8–18 mg/dl, F—8–18 mg/dl.

Table H Age, Sex and Serum Calcium Level

Sex	Age	N	Mean (mg/dl)	Range
M	20–39	1,529	10.04	9.2–10.8
M	40–59	2,009	9.91	9.0–10.8
M	60–79	382	9.82	8.9–10.7
F	20–39	1,943	9.81	8.9–10.7
F	40–59	2,355	9.82	8.8–10.8
F	60–79	590	9.89	9.1–10.7

Adapted from Cutler, 1970.
Standard Normal Value = M—9.0–10.6 mg/dl, F—9.0–10.6 mg/dl, 4.5–5.3 mEq/l.

Table I Cholesterol Levels of Seventh Decade Adults

Sex	Age	Range (mg/dl)
Males	70–79	154–314
Females	70–79	171–347

Adapted from Cutler, 1970.
Standard Normal Values: M—150–750 mg/dl, F—150–250 mg/dl.

Table J Age, Sex and Serum Creatinine Level

Sex	Age	N	Mean (mg/dl)	Range
M	20–39	1,529	1.09	0.7–1.5
M	40–59	2,009	1.12	0.8–1.5
M	60–79	382	1.17	0.7–1.6
F	20–39	1,943	0.89	0.6–1.2
F	40–59	2,355	0.95	0.6–1.3
F	60–79	590	0.99	0.6–1.4

Adapted from Cutler, 1970.
Standard Normal Value: M—0.6–1.2 mg/dl, F—0.6–1.2 mg/dl.

Table K Age and Creatinine Clearance Values of Men

Age	(N)	(Mean)
25–34	73	140.1
45–54	152	126.8
65–74	68	109.5
75–84	29	96.9

Adapted from Rowe, 1976.
Standard Normal Value: M—107–140 mg/min.

Table L Age, Sex and Fasting Glucose Level

Sex	Age	N	Mean (mg/dl)	Range
M	20–39	817	91.91	62.5–121.2
M	40–59	2380	94.66	61.1–128.2
M	60–79	520	95.16	51.8–135.4
F	20–39	265	91.40	59.5–120.7
F	40–59	561	96.08	64.6–128.0
F	60–79	268	96.35	57.8–135.2

Adapted from Wilding, Rollason, and Robinson, 1972.
Standard Normal Value: M/F—70–110 mg/dl (serum or plasma), 60–100 mg/dl (whole blood).

Table M Age, Sex and Inorganic Phosphorus Level

Sex	Age	N	Mean (mg/dl)	Range
M	20–39	817	3.53	2.3–4.8
M	40–59	2380	3.50	2.3–4.7
M	60–79	520	3.59	2.2–5.0
F	20–39	265	3.63	2.6–4.7
F	40–59	561	3.71	2.4–4.9
F	60–79	268	3.88	2.7–5.1

Adapted from Wilding, Rolloson, and Robinson, 1972.
Standard Normal Values: M—3.0–4.5 mg/dl, F—3.0–4.5 mg/dl.

Table N Age, Sex and Serum Potassium Level

Sex	Age	N	Mean (mEq/l)	Range
M	20–39	817	4.36	3.6–5.1
M	40–59	2380	4.42	3.6–5.2
M	60–79	520	4.52	3.6–5.6
F	20–39	265	4.30	3.5–5.1
F	40–59	561	4.34	3.5–5.2
F	60–79	268	4.40	3.5–5.3

Adapted from Wilding, Rolloson, and Robinson, 1972.
Standard Normal Values: M—3.8–5.0 mEq/l, F—3.8–5.0 mEq/l.

Table O Age, Sex and Total Protein Level

Sex	Age	N	Mean (gm/dl)	Range
M	20–39	1529	7.11	6.2–8.0
M	40–59	2009	6.97	6.0–7.9
M	60–79	382	6.92	6.0–7.9
F	20–39	1943	6.93	6.0–7.8
F	40–59	2355	6.87	6.0–7.8
F	60–79	590	6.83	5.9–7.8

Adapted from Cutler, 1970.
Standard Normal Values: M—6.0–7.8 gm/dl, F—6.0–7.8 gm/dl.

Table P Age, Sex and Serum Sodium Level

Sex	Age	N	Mean (mEq/l)	Range
M	20–39	817	140.51	134.6–146.4
M	40–59	2380	140.51	135.1–146.0
M	60–79	520	140.40	134.0–146.6
F	20–39	265	139.84	134.4–145.4
F	40–59	561	140.39	134.6–146.0
F	60–79	768	140.60	134.7–146.8

Adapted from Wilding, Rolloson, and Robinson, 1972.
Standard Normal Values: M—136–142 mEq/l, F—136–142 mEq/l.

Table Q Age, Sex and Uric Acid Level

Sex	Age	N	Mean (mg/dl)	Range
M	20–39	1529	5.48	3.0–7.9
M	40–59	2009	5.52	3.0–8.0
M	60–79	382	5.69	2.9–8.8
F	20–39	1943	3.84	2.0–5.7
F	40–59	2355	4.07	2.1–6.1
F	60–79	590	4.62	2.2–7.2

Adapted from Cutler, 1970.
Standard Normal Values: M—2.1–7.8 mg/dl, F—2.0–6.4 mg/dl.

Table R Oral Glucose Tolerance Test

Study[a]	Glucose dose (g)	Source of Blood[d]	Age (yr) Young	Age (yr) Old	Mean Blood Glucose[e] (mg%) 1 HR Young	1 HR Old	2 HR Young	2 HR Old	Age Effect on Glucose (condition mg% per decade life) 1 hr	2 hr
U.S. Nat. Center										
Health Stat., 1964	50	V	18–24	75–79	100	166	—	—	12	—
Welborn et al., 1969	50	V	21–29	70	86	135	—	—	10	—
Boyns et al., 1969	50	V	24	55	89	165	74	78	9	1
Nilsson et al., 1967	(50)[b]	C	20–39	60–79	111	154	—	—	11	—
Butterfield, 1966	50	C	20–29	70–79	125	194	86	121	14	7
Diabetes Survey										
Working Party, 1963	50	C	29	70	122	186	98	119	13	4
Hayner et al., 1965	100	V	16–19	70–79	100	177	—	—	13	—
Unger, 1957	100	V	18–29	50–59	—	—	99	131	—	11
Studer et al., 1969	100	C	25–34	65–74	—	—	98	127	—	7
Gerontology Research Center, 1972	(122)[c]	V	20–29	70–79	144	174	113	145	6	6

Adapted from Andres and Tobin (1977).

[a] In studies 3–6 and 8–10, glucose was ingested in the morning after an overnight fast. In studies 1, 2, and 7, subjects presented themselves for testing at various times of the day and at various time intervals after the last meal.

[b] 30 g glucose per m² surface area—50 g for man of average size.

[c] 1.75 g per kg body weight = 122 g per 70 kg man.

[d] V = antecubital venous blood; C = capillary blood.

[e] It should be stressed that these values should not be taken as the upper limits of normality. They represent mean values. Note that at 2 hours the *mean* value for the old subjects is equal to or exceeds 120 mg%, a level commonly taken to be the upper limit of normality.

Standard Normal Values: Fasting—70–110 mg/dl, 5 min—maximum of 250 mg/dl, 60 min—below 120 mg/dl, 180 min—fasting level.

191

Table S Age, Sex and Alkaline Phosphatase Level

Sex	Age	N	Mean* (KAU/dl)	Range
M	20–39	817	9.46	4.2–14.8
M	40–59	2380	9.88	4.1–15.8
M	60–79	520	9.42	2.0–16.7
F	20–39	265	7.19	2.7–11.6
F	40–59	561	8.81	2.6–16.1
F	60–79	268	10.58	3.7–17.6

Adapted from Wilding, Rollason, and Robinson, 1972.
* King-Armstrong Units (KAU).
Standard Normal Values: M/F—4.0–13.0 KAU/dl.

Table T Age, Sex and Lactate Dehydrogenase Levels

Sex*	Age	Mean (IU/l)
M	20–29	145
M	30–39	153
M	40–49	148
M	50–59	159
M	60–69	159
M	70–79	176
F	20–29	138
F	30–39	143
F	40–49	148
F	50–59	161
F	60–69	173
F	70–79	163

Adapted from Werner, 1972.
* Total sample size, combining both sexes, greater than 3000.
Standard Normal Values: M—71–207 IU/l, F—71–207 IU/l.

Table U Age, Sex, and Serum Glutamic Oxalacetic Transaminase (SGOT), Serum Glutamic Pyruvic Transaminanse (SGPT), and Serum Creatine Phosphokinase (SCPK)

Enzyme	Sex	Age	N	Mean	Range
SGOT[a,d] (u/ml)	M	20–39	1529	18.57	0.0–48.4
	M	40–59	2009	19.01	0.0–43.1
	M	60–79	382	18.75	0.2–38.1
	F	20–39	1943	14.82	3.1–26.5
	F	40–59	2355	16.24	0.0–44.8
	F	60–79	590	16.89	1.8–31.8
SGPT[b,e] (u/l)	M/F	20–45	20	17.2	6.6–27.6
	M/F	51–64	21	8.6	0.0–18.4
	M/F	65–74	28	7.3	0.0–15.3
	M/F	75–89	31	9.7	0.0–22.3
SCPK[c,f] (u/l)	—	—	—	—	—

[a] Adapted from Cutler, 1970.
[b] Adapted from Cononi, Maneti, and Benatti, 1963.
[c] Talley, 1979.
[d] Standard Normal Values: M/F—8–33 u/ml.
[e] Standard Normal Values: M/F—1–36 u/l.
[f] Standard Normal Values: M—55–170 u/l @ 37°C, F—30–135 u/l @ 37°C.

Table V Age, Percent of Urea Clearance and Specific Gravity of Urine

Age	Urea Clearance Test		Addis-Shervky Concentration Test	
	N	Percentage of Clearance of Young Males	N	Specific Gravity of Urine
40–49	20	95	8	1.0293
50–59	20	86	4	1.0287
60–69	20	82	8	1.02777
70–79	20	65	7	1.0253
80–89	20	61	11	1.0238

Adapted from Korenchersky, 1961.
Standard Normal Values: 1.016–1.022 (with normal fluid intake). Range = 1.001–1.035.

REFERENCES

Andres, R., & Tobin, J. (1977). Endocrine systems. In C. Finch & L. Hayflick (Eds.), *Handbook of the biology of aging* (pp. 357–378). New York: Van Nostrand Reinhold.

Conconi, F., Manenti, F., & Benatti, G. (1963). Behavior of some enzyme activities in plasma in normal subjects in relation to age. *Acta Vitaminologica, 17,* 33–35.

Cutler, J. (1970). Normal values for multiphasic screening blood chemistry test. In *Advances in automated analysis. Technicon International Congress, 1969* (vol. III) (pp. 67–73). White Plains, NY: Medaid, Inc.

Davidshohn, I., & Henry, J. (1974). *Todd-Sanford clinical diagnosis by laboratory methods* (15th ed.). Philadelphia: W.B. Saunders Co.

Hayes, G., & Stinson, I. (1976). Erythrocyte sedimentation rate and age. *Archives of Ophthalmology, 94,* 939–940.

Korenchevsky, V. (1961). *Physiological and pathological aging.* New York: Hafner Publishing Co.

Libow, L. (1963). Medical Investigation of the processes of aging. In J. Birren, R. Butler, S. Greenhouse, et al. (Eds.), *Human aging: A biological and behavioral study* (p. 37). Publication Number (HSM) 71-9051. Washington, DC: United States Government Printing Office.

Meakawa, T. (1976). Hematologic diseases. In F. Sternberg (Ed.), *Cowdry's the care of the geriatric patient* (pp. 152–156). St. Louis: C.V. Mosby Co.

Rowe, J. (1976). The effect of age on creatinine clearance in men: A cross sectional and logitudinal study. *Journal of Gerontology, 31,* 155–163.

Shapleigh, J., Mayes, S., & Moore, C. (1952). Hematologic values in the aged. *Journal of Gerontology, 7,* 207–219.

Talley, L. (1979). Laboratory values. In D. Carnevali & M. Patrick (Eds.), *Nursing management for the elderly* (pp. 81–110). Philadelphia: Lippincott Co. Werner, M. (1970). Influence of sex and age on the normal range of eleven serum constituents. *Zeitschrift fur Klinische Chemie und Klinische Biochemie, 8,* 105–115.

Wilding, P., Rollason, J., & Robinson, D. (1972). Patterns of change for various biochemical constituents detected in well population screening. *Clinica Chimica Acta, 41,* 375–387.

Index

A

Activity theory of aging, 17
Activity therapy, in
    psychotherapy, 130
Acute disease, in elderly, 26
Acute intermittent porphyria, 78
Acute organic mental syndrome,
    111–112, 119. *See also*
    Organic mental syndrome
Adrenal glands, 44–45
Advocacy groups, for elderly, 177
Age
  biological, 6
  chronological, 5–6
  functional, 7
  legal, 5–6
  old, definition of, 5
  psychological, 6–7
  sociological, 6
Aging
  and cardiovascular system, 36–
    38
  definitions of, 1–9
  and disease, 25–27
  and endocrine system, 43–45
  and gastrointestinal system, 40–
    42
  and genitourinary system, 38–40
  and hematopoietic system, 40
  and integumentary system, 41

---

t = table

and musculoskeletal system,
    45–46
and nervous system, 46–48
"normal," 7–8, 28–29
research on, 180
and respiratory system, 40–41
theories of, 11–19
  cellular, 15–17
  hereditary, 11–13
  physiological, 13–15
  psychosocial, 17–19
Alcoholism, 85–86
Alertness, 98
Alkaline phosphatase, 185, 191*t*
Anemia, 84–85
Anesthesia, and drug use, 87
Antianxiety agents, 156–159
Antibodies, of autoimmune
    system, 15
Anticholinergic activity, 159–161,
    163
Antidepressant agents, 159–161
Antihistamines, 153
Antipsychotic agents, 161–164
  antiparkinson drugs, 162–163
  thioridazine, 161
Antipyrine, 146
Anxiety, and antianxiety agents,
    156–159
Aorta, 37–38. *See also*
    Cardiovascular system
Aphasia, 81, 115
Appearance, in assessment of
    mental processes, 61–62

Psychotropic drug intervention
(continued)
 antidepressant agents, 159–161
 antipsychotic agents, 161–164
 sedatives, 152–156
Pulmonary embolic disease, 77
Pyridoxine deficiency, 85

R

RNA synthesis impairment, 16
Race, effect of on aging, 28
Reality, distortion of. *See*
 Psychosis
Reality orientation, in
 psychotherapy, 130–131
Reflexes, in chronic organic
 mental syndrome, 114–115
Reminiscence, in psychotherapy,
 131, 134
Remotivation, in psychotherapy,
 131
Renal function, 39
 disorders, 73–75
 and excretion, of drugs, 146–148
Reproductive system, and aging,
 11, 12, 39–40
Resocialization-remotivation, in
 psychotherapy, 131
Respiratory system
 age-related changes in, 40–41
 disease of, 76–77
Response patterns, of elderly, 82

S

Sedatives, 152–156
 antihistamines, 153
 benzodiazepines, 153–156
Senile dementia. *See* Organic
 mental syndrome
Senior centers, 173–174
Sensorium, disorders of, 63–64

Sensory stimulation, in
 psychotherapy, 129–130,
 134
Sexual activity, of elderly, 24
Skin, 41
Sleep disorders, treatment of,
 153–156
Small intestine, and drug
 absorption, 140–141
Smoking, and life expectancy, 30t.
Snouting, and chronic organic
 mental syndrome, 115
Social activity, of elderly, 17
Social history, and assessment of
 mental processes, 61
Social interaction of elderly, 17
Social learning approaches, 133–
 134
Socioeconomic status, and
 disease, 26
Sociological age, 6
Sociotherapeutic interventions,
 171–182
 and advocacy, 177
 and consumerism, 177–178
 day care, 173
 and education, 176
 and food services, 174
 and government, role of, 179–
 180
 and home health care, 175–176
 and homemaker services, 175
 and peer counseling, 176–177
 senior centers, 173–174
 and transportation, 174
Spatial perception, in chronic
 organic mental syndrome,
 116
Speech
 and assessment of mental
 processes, 62, 64
 in chronic organic mental
 syndrome, 115